RECOVERY GROUPS

Recovery Groups

A GUIDE TO CREATING, LEADING, AND WORKING WITH GROUPS FOR ADDICTIONS AND MENTAL HEALTH CONDITIONS

By Linda Farris Kurtz

OXFORD
UNIVERSITY PRESS

OXFORD
UNIVERSITY PRESS

Oxford University Press is a department of the University of Oxford. It furthers the University's objective of excellence in research, scholarship, and education by publishing worldwide.

Oxford New York
Auckland Cape Town Dar es Salaam Hong Kong Karachi
Kuala Lumpur Madrid Melbourne Mexico City Nairobi
New Delhi Shanghai Taipei Toronto

With offices in
Argentina Austria Brazil Chile Czech Republic France Greece
Guatemala Hungary Italy Japan Poland Portugal Singapore
South Korea Switzerland Thailand Turkey Ukraine Vietnam

Oxford is a registered trademark of Oxford University Press in the UK and certain other countries.

Published in the United States of America by
Oxford University Press
198 Madison Avenue, New York, NY 10016

A copy of this book's Catalog-in-Publication Data is on file with the Library of Congress
ISBN 978–0–19–936297–4

To Ernest Kurtz

Contents

PART 2

Foreword

RECENT DECADES STAND as a watershed era in the history of recovery as an organizing construct for addiction treatment and mental health services in the United States and other countries. Recovery mutual-aid groups are growing exponentially, as evidenced by their number, size, philosophical diversification, and increased specialization. New recovery-support institutions—grass-roots recovery community organizations, centers, clubhouses, cafes, residences, schools, industries, and ministries—continue to spread. Advocacy movements organized by and for people in recovery are coming of age and mobilizing numbers of people that would have been unthinkable only a few years ago. Approaches to professional treatment are being extended from models of acute stabilization and palliative care to assertive models of long-term personal and family recovery. Representation of people in recovery is growing at all levels within behavioral health systems, with peer recovery-support services flourishing amid growing calls to create recovery-oriented systems of care. The vision and reality of long-term recovery are reshaping behavioral health policies, programs, and front-line service practices. If there is what could be called an age of recovery, we are clearly entering it.

And if there is a ground zero from which this recovery revolution is unfolding, it is clearly the critical mass that has been reached through the growth of recovery mutual-aid groups. The increased professionalization and commercialization of addiction treatment and mental health services in the mid-twentieth century led to a disconnection between grass-roots communities of recovery and professional systems of care. That disconnection is now being reversed, but professional caregivers are ill prepared for this new world. Education of physicians, nurses, psychologists, social workers, addiction counselors, mental health counselors, and other allied professionals has provided little training on the prevalence, pathways, processes, and stages of long-term personal and family recovery and even less about the history, organization, culture, and etiquette of secular, spiritual, and religious recovery mutual-aid organizations. What is needed is a history- and science-informed primer on the nature of such groups and how professionals can collaborate with these groups without harming them in the process. Linda Kurtz's latest contribution, *Recovery Groups*, provides just such a primer.

Recovery Groups outlines the history of recovery mutual-aid groups, explores the core characteristics that distinguish them from professional care, and profiles some of the major recovery mutual-aid groups in the United States. Kurtz further reviews research on the major mechanisms of change that operate within these groups and offers concrete guidance on how service professionals can facilitate collaboration with and effective referrals to these resources. Of particular note is the closing chapter on the growing phenomenon of virtual recovery—the management of personal recovery through support garnered from online support groups and related online communications. A day may come sooner than any could predict when more people will be involved in Internet-based recovery support than in face-to-face recovery-support meetings. *Recovery Groups* offers a window into this future by exploring both the potential and the risks associated with Internet-based mutual aid.

Recovery Groups is well conceived, well researched, and well written. It will find a wide and appreciative audience among all those interested in behavioral health problems and solutions. I suspect it will become the primer for training behavioral health professionals for years to come. Professionals are at their best when they enter communities of recovery from a position of curiosity, respect, and humility—as inquiring students rather than as teachers. The best way to learn about recovery mutual-aid groups is the direct experience of conversing with people in recovery and observing open meetings, but preparation, such as reading *Recovery Groups*, will enrich such experiences.

The foundational scales of orientation within behavioral healthcare are tipping from a focus on pathology and intervention technologies to a focus on the programs and processes of long-term recovery. The following pages constitute a needed guidebook to these cultures of recovery.

WILLIAM L. WHITE

AUTHOR, *Slaying the Dragon: The History of Addiction Treatment and Recovery in America*

Preface

I BEGAN MY social work career in 1958 at the age of nineteen, when I was a social work aide at Topeka State Hospital in Kansas. My job was to link stabilized patients on the third floor of the west side of the Eastman Building with board-and-care homes in town. These were elderly patients whose massive records showed they had been incarcerated and sterilized as young men and had lived their entire lives in the hospital. The fact that they were on the third floor on that side of the building meant that they were stable enough to work at a job on the grounds of the hospital and therefore also able to live in the community, at least theoretically.

This scene was being enacted in every building at Topeka State—a college student, wanting a career in social work, making connections for stabilized patients to enter community placements. We may have been ahead of our time, performing deinstitutionalization in the 1950s.

This was our procedure: Staff identified a patient and referred him to me. I filled out a long form, talked with the patient, and contacted the family to tell them their son or brother was ready to be discharged. I then identified a board-and-care home where the patient might go. The board-and-care homes had been preselected and licensed by the county welfare office. Only one of my cases had family who still wanted him back. They lived on a farm, and he was able to go home and do the same job he had been doing at the hospital for many years, working in the fields.

The Eastman Building had an intake floor, an acute treatment floor, and an open ward for the newer patients to begin reentering the outside world. New entries did not remain in the hospital as the older generation of patients had done, before tranquilizers. There were two other floors in the Eastman Building, locked wards where no female was allowed. Looking in through the tiny window of one of these, one saw a large number of elderly men pacing about and presumably violent, at least dangerous to be around. This is my memory; someone else might remember it differently. Despite the gruesome conditions for patients, I liked working there and, at least at times in later years, would have returned.

Much later in my career, in 1974, I encountered Alcoholics Anonymous for the first time when I helped implement a community residential program in the county where I worked outside Atlanta, Georgia. The community program was the outcome of local efforts by AA members acting on their own; the state mental health system helped the program by allocating supportive living funds for their residents. My work with this program convinced me that the mental health field needed a self-help network like AA. I chose the topic for a doctoral dissertation and continued along the same research path for the rest of my career as an academic in social work. I realize now that there will probably never be another mutual-aid network like AA that can offer recovering persons the availability of meetings almost around the clock and a social world that can so absorb them that they can have virtually no contact with a former network of drinkers unless they really want to. There are many reasons it's good that AA is out there, but one large one is to have an ideal for which to strive.

Writing this book led me to the literature on several programs in which mutual help is used to provide housing, employment, and social relationships for people with psychiatric disabilities. My intention in writing this book was to rewrite and reimagine my 1997 textbook on self-help and support groups. I have done that, but I've also placed my presentation of these groups within the concept of the recovery model and extended the focus into advocacy groups and supportive recovery programs such as Fountain House.

Part II of this book explores what is known about working with, creating, and leading self-help and support groups for mental health and for addiction. Part III branches out away from the inner workings of reform-oriented supportive kinds of groups and into the broader community of groups and services that build on self-help. It examines mutual-support and person-initiated recovery following acute care, noting how the dynamics of groups impel members to change the community and the array of services it offers. It considers community approaches to changing social policy and to changing the environment where people go to continue their recovery. Finally, it surveys life online and how the computer can bring a person to a meeting where he or she gains acceptance, support, and advice at any time of the day or night.

As I say in the conclusion to the book, mental health services seem to be decreasing as more and more people need them. Community mutual-aid groups, which cost very little, can take up some of the slack and offer people in recovery a place to go for social relationships and emotional support. And that's no small thing.

RECOVERY GROUPS

1

INTRODUCTION

THIS VOLUME IS meant to guide practitioners, members, agency directors, and policy makers at all levels in making groups work as a force for meeting recovery goals: adjustment to life without chemicals, finding work and shelter, coping with relationships, developing friendships, living with symptoms, and many others. Most groups either have an appointed leader or share leadership roles among members. The suggestions contained here can apply to any of these roles and situations, any type of support or mutual-help group, and any type of leader, whether peer or professional.

The book is about recovery for people with mental health conditions and addictions. It is divided into three parts. Part I begins with chapter 2 and an overview of the recovery model and how it has developed in both sectors of service. Chapter 3 introduces the reader to four types of groups, how they differ, and when to form one type of group or the other. It also familiarizes the reader with the self-help ethos and the two seminal characteristics of self-help: the helper therapy principle and experiential knowledge. Chapter 4 introduces a few of the major groups for addictions, mental health conditions, and people who cope with both. The groups profiled represent only a few of the self-help associations in the country and do not describe smaller, local support groups or consumer-run programs.

Part II focuses on working with groups. Chapter 5 discusses the role of the practitioner (usually a staff person in a treatment agency) who links individuals with independent self-help groups. It begins by telling the stories of some of the larger fellowships' founders. It goes on to address how you can help a recovery group get started and, more important, how you can link people to a group in such a way that you know they attended and can monitor the results. How do you help a group without affecting its self-help character?

Chapter 6 focuses on support groups (as opposed to larger, more complex self-help, mutual-aid groups) and how a professional or lay leader goes about starting a support group, facilitating a meeting, and maintaining membership. Understanding the stages of group development gives direction for support group facilitation. The chapter concludes with a discussion of typical problems encountered in support groups.

Chapter 7 delves further into the factors that help people get support, use information, and learn to use a method of recovery. Drawing on some of Irving Yalom's list of therapeutic factors in therapy groups, it applies them to support and mutual-help groups and examines how a leader or a member can enhance these processes within the group. It continues with a look at what self-help and support group research reveals about helping factors and concludes with an examination of some of the identified unhelpful characteristics that groups acquire, offering suggestions on how to prevent or eliminate them.

Chapter 8 examines the concept of group climate, how it is measured, and typical climates found in self-help and support groups. It discusses methods of moderating a group climate to bring it closer to an ideal. The chapter then explains group worldviews, those beliefs and teachings that the group has developed to help its members acquire new understandings of their experience so that they can move forward. It examines organizational structure, offering suggestions for possible structural modifications.

Chapter 9 considers how some people are natural joiners while others prefer not to affiliate themselves with groups. It examines change-readiness and stages of group affiliation and discusses "old-timers" (long-term members) and why they are important to a group.

Chapter 10 presents in-depth looks at examples of various types of groups: a twelve-step group, Al-Anon Family Groups; an older established mental-health-oriented group, Recovery International; a newer association for people with schizophrenia and related disorders, Schizophrenics Anonymous; and a dual recovery group for people with both psychiatric disorders and drug and alcohol dependence, Dual Recovery Anonymous. This chapter is intended to clarify how some groups have adopted AA's Twelve Steps and Twelve Traditions almost verbatim and how others have borrowed some of the AA program's principles and left out others. One association, Recovery International, is included to show how a self-help group with a complex program evolved without using the steps and traditions.

Part III examines mutual aid in society, showing how AA influenced the development of the National Council on Alcoholism and Drug Dependency despite its traditions advocating anonymity. Chapter 11 focuses specifically on how apolitical organizations such as twelve-step groups find ways to influence policy without bringing controversial issues into the group process. It highlights the newer Faces & Voices Association of Recovery Community Organizations, discusses in detail the National Alliance on Mental Illness, and treats mental health consumer/survivor advocacy groups and coalitions.

Chapter 12 examines three nationwide agencies that deliver consumer-run (or partially consumer-run) services in psychiatric and addiction fields using mutual-help methods: Fairweather Lodge, Oxford Houses, and the Fountain House working community model. This chapter is included to show how self-help and mutual aid can exist as part of a larger service system and how the system can change its goals for a consumer from symptom management to life transformation.

Chapter 13 discusses online groups. Most self-help associations in the mental health and addiction fields offer both face-to-face groups and online groups. The chapter examines a variety of methods used to supply members and potential members with help and support in the cyber-world.

The conclusion comes back to the original intention of this book: encouraging the reader to appreciate, value, and use community self-help and support groups, the indispensable community recovery groups that can help construct meaningful existence for people who may not have completely benefited from professional treatment or, even more, who may not have had such help available at all.

1

[R]ecovery is an attitude, a stance, and a way of approaching the day's challenges. It is a self-directed process of reclaiming meaning and purpose in life.
DEEGAN (2005, p. 67)

2

THE RECOVERY APPROACH IN MENTAL HEALTH AND ADDICTION

RECOVERING ALCOHOLICS ATTEND meetings of Alcoholics Anonymous (AA). At least, that's the expectation. Actually, some convalescing alcoholics don't go to meetings at all. I knew a man many years ago who was a powerful and admired citizen despite the fact that he drank too much. His doctor told him, "You are going to die if you don't stop drinking." The man stopped. He let it be known that he had stopped drinking but was not an alcoholic because he did not have to "go to meetings," that is, AA. He just stopped. Some said he wasn't really an alcoholic; others called him a "dry drunk" (still thinking like an alcoholic). He was that type of heavy drinker whom E. M. Jelinek, who is famous for the disease concept of alcoholism, called the "beta alcoholic"—the one who suffers physical, but not psychological, harm from heavy alcohol use (Jelinek, 1960). It's as if the alcohol made no impression on his brain, only the rest of his body. This does not mean that his condition was not serious or that he was not the "real deal." He was an alcoholic, and he was endangering his life just as much as someone who drinks and drives endangers his life and the lives of others or as much as the alcoholic who loses everything as a result of drinking.

Whatever you think about that man, he did stop drinking, on his own, in his own way. Many people diagnosed with addictive or mental disorder recover that way (Corrigan & Ralph, 2005), but that does not mean anyone can do it. For some people, symptoms of addiction or mental health problems are too much for them to handle alone. Some have no support system, or what they have doesn't help, so those individuals don't make it without the aid of treatment programs and recovery groups. What is the elusive element that makes success come easily to some and escapes others? Robert Granfield and William Cloud's (1999) research on "self-remitters," people who recover from alcoholism without either treatment or a recovery group such as AA, found that such individuals possess high degrees of "recovery capital," which means having resources "such as education, occupational skills, financial stability, and supportive families and friends" (p. 163). The man mentioned above had all those assets in abundance. Most people in difficulty try to overcome it first with the resources they already have, but when those fail, treatment and recovery groups come to the rescue. People recuperating from psychological or addiction-related disabilities need recovery capital, the acquisition of which is one of the primary goals of the recovery approach to service.

This book is about recovery groups, not just for alcoholics but also for drug users and people affected by mental health conditions. Public policy experts, researchers, and clinicians agree that there is a process called recovery that goes beyond the first few weeks of treatment and may go on for many years as people struggle with chronic conditions brought on by chemicals, high levels of stress, brain abnormalities, or all three. Pressure by ex-patient groups and recovering addicts has spawned a philosophy of recovery and a paradigmatic shift that influence the mental health sector and the separate, but similar, addiction sector of public health care. Before focusing on recovery groups, this chapter will briefly summarize how the recovery approach came about in the two separate fields of service and highlight how recovery groups sparked the origins of the recovery movement in both fields and have become a part of the methodology of recovery care.

First, let's briefly consider how the brain is affected in mental and addictive disorders and thus why the individual in recovery may need extended support. Both mental health and addictive conditions are heavily stigmatized. People with mental health problems are thought to be dangerous and strange, so much so that those who can do so hide the condition in fear of being ostracized. Alcoholics and other addicts are thought to be weak and self-indulgent people who use their chosen drugs in spite of negative consequences to themselves and others and despite numerous efforts to help them. Few people really understand the mental processes that lead to and reinforce addiction and mental health conditions. In addition, few treatment providers realize how long it can take to recover successfully.

Common explanations of both psychiatric disorder and addiction hold that these conditions are the product of brain abnormality. This is particularly applicable to addiction wherein a substance crosses the blood-brain barrier repeatedly and affects the brain in such a way as to change it. These changes can result in feelings of irresistible pleasure when using the substance, which reinforces additional use. They can also produce, over time, intolerable sensations of anxiety that can only be eased by additional consumption of the substance. Both of these factors lead to "the overpowering motivational strength and decreased ability to control the desire to obtain drugs" (Kalivas & Volkow, 2005, p. 1403). This helps to explain why chronic alcoholism and other drug use are so intractable and require extended periods of supported recovery management.

In regard to mental illnesses, many think of them as diseases of the brain; others contend that this understanding is flawed (Grohol, 2011). Whatever the case, for some people who have mental health conditions, there are factors affecting brain functions that make returning to previous functioning difficult and thus demand extended community support, at least until such time as the neuroplasticity of the brain allows it to regenerate necessary functions (Doidge, 2007).

THE PARADIGM SHIFT FROM MEDICAL MODEL TO RECOVERY MODEL

William White and Ernest Kurtz (2006) reviewed the evolution of treatment paradigms in the alcoholism and drug treatment field. All previous models, they noted, began with some concept of the cause of the disorder: sin, spiritual despair, criminality, mental illness/disease, psychological malfunction, or sociocultural influences. From these positions come various modes of intervention, all of which have elicited scientific research and debate. The authors and others proposed a recovery model that does not come from theories of causation but instead is based on the experiences of successful recovery drawn from the millions who have achieved it.

The path to the recovery treatment paradigm for addictions goes back to the founding of AA in 1935 and, later, the Minnesota Model articulated and implemented by Dan Anderson at Hazelden in Center City, Minnesota, in the 1950s (Anderson, McGovern, & DuPont, 1999). The Minnesota Model included a role for peer helpers and involved patients in AA while they were still in treatment. Anderson believed the success of the Minnesota Model came from infusing the treatment program with the spirit of mutual help found in AA (Anderson et al., 1999; Spicer, 1993). This prototype formed the basis of inpatient and outpatient treatment throughout this country and the world for many decades. The often haphazard affiliation with AA after treatment would be the focus of much research, at first in an effort to decide which was better, treatment or AA (Humphreys, 2004). As time went on, research showed that both were better than one or the other, and efforts to link patients to AA during and after treatment increased. Yet the connection between treatment program and community mutual aid was often inadequate, and many consumers dropped by the wayside once they were discharged from short-term treatment. Recognition of the importance of continuing recovery in a self-help environment too often failed to translate into action. Recovery for many does not mean return to life as it existed before the addiction; it means being in a process of taking each day at a time and practicing principles of a sober life over a long period. Thus, this early effort to connect discharged patients to the mutual-helping community became one of the foundation stones of today's recovery approach in addiction treatment.

In the mental health field, recovery is "addressed in the context of a social disability paradigm rather than a medical one" (Walsh, 2013, p. 14). Recovery can mean full recovery, or it may mean partial recovery (Davidson, Tondora, Lawless, O'Connell, & Rowe, 2009). The gradual shift from multiple causation theories to peer-supportive recovery methods focused less on biological and psychodynamic theories and more on common elements after acute treatment ends. The shift in the mental health sector has been much more gradual and less obvious than the alcohol treatment transition to the Minnesota Model. Historically, aftercare planning under the medical model involved making sure the patient had prescriptions for medications, appointments for follow-up psychiatric treatment, and family support. That planning did not include linkages to a self-help community and often not to employment or housing so that recovery could progress along lines that meant more than symptom removal.

Early in my social work career (in the 1960s and '70s), I worked on an inpatient unit in a mental health institute that housed an alcohol treatment program in a separate building. I experienced culture shock when I spent a week of training in that other building while I was still working in adult psychiatry. Multidisciplinary evaluations, formal therapy sessions, and staff rounds followed set patterns on the mental health treatment unit. In the alcohol program, peer helpers were part of the staff and ran staff meetings with frequent references to AA slogans, didactic lectures took the place of psychotherapy, and the spirit of AA overflowed in the old, run-down mansion that housed the program. The two models of care could not have been more different. Those differences and others have put barriers between the two service sectors that make integrated care difficult to this day (White & Davidson, 2006a, 2006b). Table 2.1 shows that the seeds of recovery methods in both fields began at the same time (the late 1930s to the early 1950s), but only in the addiction treatment sector does its version of the recovery model dominate the field.

I thought then that mental health consumers would benefit from something similar to the AA-modeled programs in alcohol treatment, but from my vantage point in the state of Georgia, I did not see it happening in the 1970s and '80s. In the mental health field, the roots of peer support back in the late 1970s seemed to emerge from the mental health consumer movement, especially from Judy Chamberlin. Her 1978 book, *On Our Own: Patient Controlled Alternatives to Mental Health Care*, was one of the first to articulate protests and calls to action by and on behalf of people who were being treated in psychiatric institutions. The mental patients liberation

TABLE 2.1
EVOLUTION OF RECOVERY MODEL IN MENTAL HEALTH AND ADDICTION TREATMENT SERVICE SECTORS

	Mental Health Treatment Sector	Addiction Treatment Sector
Origin	1948 Fountain House	1952 Minnesota Model
Place	New York, NY	Center City, MN
Self-help group influence	Recovery, Inc., 1937 We Are Not Alone, 1944	Alcoholics Anonymous, 1935 Narcotics Anonymous, 1953
Original treatment paradigm	Custodial care/no treatment	Custodial care/no treatment
Public attitude	Hopeless	Hopeless
Recent paradigms of care	Medical (mental illness is an incurable brain disease) Social (psychiatric rehabilitation, clubhouse) Recovery paradigm, 2003	Pathology paradigm (alcoholism is an incurable disease) Intervention paradigm (short-term, acute care) Recovery paradigm, 2003
Evolving public policy	Community mental health centers, 1963–65 Community Support Program, 1977 New Freedom Commission on Mental Health, 2003	1970 Hughes Act[1] (publicly supported intervention and treatment) New Freedom Commission on Mental Health, 2003
Goals of recovery-oriented treatment	Symptom accommodation Support for jobs, housing, recreation, and socialization	Abstinence—reduction in use—sober living Sustained recovery management—connection to community of recovery

[1] Comprehensive Alcohol Abuse and Alcoholism Prevention, Treatment, and Rehabilitation Act of 1970.

movement, now thought of as the mental health consumer/survivor movement, exerted pressure from 1970 to 2000 to influence mental health policy in the United States. Finally, the President's New Freedom Commission on Mental Health in 2003 came out with policy approaches to include and empower mental health consumers. This policy has influenced the use of self-help methods and certification and employment of peer specialists as a means of combating the severe shortage of mental health professionals and mental health services in the years following the report.

However, self-help efforts by ex-patients as early as 1944 also had a lasting impact on services for people with mental health conditions and on the current emergence of recovery methods in the field. In fact, those efforts stemmed in part from first-hand experience with AA at Rockland State Hospital in New York State (Anderson, 1998; Karlsson, 2013).

The recovery paradigm in mental health arose in 1948 with the founding of Fountain House, the first clubhouse for people with psychiatric disabilities (Anderson, 1998; Doyle, Lanoil, & Dudek, 2013). Psychosocial rehabilitation spread to Chicago in 1959. Jerry Dincin, who worked first at Fountain House, transformed the small program Thresholds into the oldest and largest mental health agency in the state of Illinois using Fountain House principles. More offshoots of the clubhouse model followed in the 1960s and '70s, and along with them came the recognition in many major cities that a disability model fit well with the protracted nature of mental health conditions (Stanhope & Solomon, 2013; Walsh, 2013).

As table 2.1 displays, both public mental health and addiction services originated out of the practice of a custodial care model suffused with hopelessness over the potential for recovery among the people with severe mental conditions and the "skid row" alcoholics of the time. The mental health medical model addressed a different, well-off, less severely ill population and anchored those methods and centers of operation firmly in the public eye and in practice. For example, the Menninger Clinic in Topeka, Kansas, treated acute cases of mental illness with the latest psychodynamic methods during those same years of custodial care for "hopeless" cases. The Menninger Clinic also treated alcoholics with the same psychodynamic methods. Well-off, less severely impaired addicts received a variety of noncustodial, medical model treatment approaches. But the wealthy alcoholics who received this care were too few in number to generate techniques widely accepted by the professions and the public. Thus, the seeds of the recovery model in both service sectors occurred at roughly the same time in history but spread widely only in the addiction sector, where peer helpers became accepted and entrenched.

Peer supports in the addictions field were rooted in mutual-aid groups, best exemplified by twelve-step programs, and became standard in almost all existing treatment settings. Twelve-step groups, especially in those early days, also harbored a generally well-concealed antiprofessional bias, but their approach took no formal positions on "outside issues" (Kurtz, 1984). The twelve-step model applied to mental health, Emotions Anonymous, for example, fit a sociological classification of "conservative, pro-mental health system groups," along with other more individual reform groups such as Recovery, Inc. (Emerick, 1991). None of the self-help mental health groups of the 1970s has had the same widespread influence on clinical care that AA had on addiction treatment in the latter part of the twentieth century. Despite that, the very small mutual-support group We Are Not Alone (WANA), a self-help group formed by ex-patients at Rockland State Hospital in New York State, began a program in New York City that would potentially transform public mental health care in the next century.

Before that happened, public policy makers in 1963 and 1965 passed the Community Mental Health Centers Acts and Amendments, which set up the nationwide system of outpatient care for the mentally ill in preparation for the deinstitutionalization of state hospitals. Inadequate to the task of helping severely mentally ill people, most mental health centers resembled outpatient services for those less impaired and not for those with serious mental health conditions. This difficult transition and pressure from the consumer movement spawned the Community Support Program of the 1970s, which led eventually to social programs instead of the medical model paradigms of the 1960s. But it would be twenty-six more years before the New Freedom Commission on Mental Health pointed the mental health field toward a recovery model. Meanwhile, the 1970 Hughes Act allocated funds for developing alcoholism and drug treatment along with the community mental health centers. Most of these public alcohol programs adhered to the twelve-step facilitation approaches used in private treatment centers, almost all of which followed the Minnesota Model.

The consumer survivor movement began in the 1970s with a radical activist membership that called itself the antipsychiatry movement. Its militant focus decreased in the 1980s. Coalitions of former mental patients formed around the country and began pressing for consumer-run programs that were eventually funded by the federal government's Community Support Program. Protection and advocacy offices were formed in states to promulgate rules about consumer rights and to defend consumers who had grievances with the system. More recently, consumers have been hired as peer specialists. Community mental health programs have begun supporting clubhouses and other psychosocial rehabilitation services, and the National Mental Health Consumers' Self-Help Clearinghouse formed a peer-run technical assistance center.

The clubhouses that formed after Fountain House inspired a new conceptual model of care: psychiatric rehabilitation. Although clubhouses have not been conceived as a type of self-help organization, much of the self-help philosophy of WANA continued with the clubhouse model as it has evolved in Fountain House, the original (Borkman, 2013). Because leadership positions are not filled by peer (recovering) administrators, clubhouses do not fit strict definitions of self-help organizations but rather are a hybrid type of association in which the mid-level of governance gives power and authority to members and restricts the power of the professionals at the top (Borkman, 2013). Brenda's story (see box 2.1) shows how this affected her experience.

BOX 2.1
BRENDA'S STORY

People were gesturing at me by waving their hands around, pointing their fingers, crossing their arms. What messages were they trying to give me? What did they expect me to do in response to their gestures? Everyone was gesturing. My family, people at work, people on the street, and even people on TV. How did the people on TV know what I was thinking? Unsolvable problems that kept me awake at night and fearful during the day. At age forty-one, I didn't understand the world anymore. I asked my brother whether we were currently in heaven or in hell on a sunny day in June, after going to his house for a visit. He got a very concerned look on his face and asked me to get in his car, which I was reluctant to do because my paranoid thoughts told me it was dangerous to trust anyone else, even family members. My sister-in-law convinced me to get in the car, and off we went to my parents' house, where they climbed in my brother's car with us, and we drove to the hospital emergency room. There, the nurse ushered us into an exam room, where I got up on the bed. I didn't really understand what was happening to me. A social worker came in at what seemed like midnight to me. He introduced himself as Matthew. I assumed he was the Matthew of the Bible who wrote one of the gospels, and I asked him if we were in heaven. Matthew disappeared after talking with me for about two minutes. He told me that I needed to move to another building where they would take care of me. What did that mean? More people gesturing at me? Thus began my first hospitalization for mental illness.

They called it bipolar disorder at first. After the third hospitalization in less than two years, it became schizoaffective disorder. I thought that by going to college for psychology and social work, I had made myself immune to the mental illness that runs in my family. I thought that by age thirty, I had dodged that bullet, because most people get sick with mental illness while in their twenties. It simply couldn't be true that I had made it to my forties and then gotten sick. I should have been grateful that it happened later in life, because, unlike others, I had worked in a successful career path and established myself as an independent adult with a house, car, pets, friends, travel. Refusing to recognize the need for medication despite my education and having worked in mental health for a few years, I lost several jobs, a house, my good financial standing, and, most painfully, my pets, a dog and two cats.

Fifth hospitalization under a ninety-day commitment by court order was the charm that made me realize that I needed my medication to stay well so that I would not keep losing control of my life and having other people take things from me like my freedom from locked mental health treatment wards and my car keys. The latter because I had driven to Canada one time and seven hundred miles away to Ocean City, Maryland, another time while psychotic and trying to escape my demons. I was also homeless, because my parents wanted to sell their house that I was living in, so I couldn't go back to it after I got out of the hospital. Indigent, no job, no insurance, on the verge of bankruptcy, I had paid a high price for my stubbornness and refusal to take my medication. My only defense is that I was afraid to take the medication that my psychiatrist had given me, because there were special messages on the side of the sample packages meant just for me that someone was trying to train me or control me for some evil purpose. It took over a year of staying on medications before my thinking straightened out and I wasn't afraid to take them.

Besides the medication, other factors were critical to my recovery, including time spent at a clubhouse in Fort Wayne called Carriage House. As part of my ninety-day commitment, I transferred from the hospital to a residential treatment program or halfway house, where we were required to go to mental health programs during the day. I had a choice of a traditional day treatment program at the local community mental health center or the clubhouse. After trying both, I chose the clubhouse. Carriage House is a warm and wonderful, safe, and inviting place where respect is in abundance and healing can begin. The program is located in a huge former farmhouse that is historic and renovated to fit the needs of the clubhouse. Why did I love the Carriage House and begin to heal there? For several reasons. First and foremost, caffeinated coffee was available for twenty-five cents. All the other mental health treatment programs and hospitals I had been at had no coffee or decaf coffee only. I was a lifelong coffee drinker; decaf just wouldn't cut it. Part of what helped me and helps people with mental illnesses recover is that they can get back to "normal"—normal life that existed before getting sick. Work, school, driving a car, real coffee. Such a small thing but a very important one to me. I also loved the clubhouse because it was impossible to tell who were the staff and who were the clients. This is by design. It definitely felt very respectful not to have the usual staff and patient differences that create barriers to communications and a lack of equality at a time when self-esteems are fragile and need to be rebuilt. Even though intellectually I knew it was for my own good, it felt bad to be behind locked doors in a place where staff had big key rings jangling on their nurses' uniforms. The clubhouse didn't have private staff offices or locked doors. Even the executive director had a desk in the middle of one of the activity rooms. The only

(*Continued*)

BOX 2.1 CONTINUED

way I could figure out who the staff were (because it didn't seem polite to ask) was that often they were in a facilitating position, helping to get activities started, but they empowered the clubhouse members to do as much as they could independently.

When I was at Carriage House, I had several options to occupy my time. I chose to do some computer work, which involved doing some bookkeeping and attendance for the clubhouse to keep records so that they could get funding from Medicare and Medicaid to help pay for the program. This was real work and important work that in a different facility most certainly would have been done by paid staff. It felt good and empowering to be doing something important and useful. That helped with my recovery more than most other treatment modalities, with the exception of medication.

Currently, I am working part-time as the executive director of a small nonprofit organization. Working is not easy, but my schedule is flexible, so that helps. I live in my own house with my three cats. I am well and have not been hospitalized since 2007, seven years ago. I receive medication and counseling from a local community mental health center. Life is good, and I am grateful that there is effective treatment available in all formats, including the clubhouse, which helped me the most.

RECOVERY PHILOSOPHY

Walsh (2013) identifies four fundamental values in the mental health recovery philosophy: hope as a catalyst of the recovery process; self-direction in controlling the path to recovery; individualized choices based on the unique strengths, needs, preferences, and cultural background of the individual; and empowerment to choose from a range of recovery options. The philosophy rests on a fundamental belief that recovery is possible, a fact not recognized in the past. It fosters improvement in four life domains: housing, work, relationships, and recreation. Recovery comes from creating a productive life in which mental health challenges are only one part of a person's identity. People with mental health conditions may continue to experience symptoms, but relief from them is not the primary goal, as it is in a medical model. Instead, consumers must adapt to the symptoms while setting personal goals for living with the disability (Stanhope & Solomon, 2013). An element in this approach to mental health disability is the use of peer helpers.

Although the addiction treatment field has integrated peer support in its basic model of services for sixty years, it long remained also mired in an acute treatment model lasting twenty-eight or fewer days. Linkages to local communities of recovery received more lip service than serious effort. A recovery philosophy in the field of addiction now recognizes that addiction is a chronic condition that can require many years of effort before sustained recovery is achieved. A dominant belief of the recovery concept in the addictions arena, therefore, posits that recovery takes place over a long time within a community of supports, many of which come from AA, NA, or other self-help groups, such as Secular Organization for Sobriety (see chapter 3). These supports include access to needed acute care, along with sustained support from peers both in groups and from individuals. Follow-up care takes place in an environment that provides housing, employment, social supports, and recreation. Acute care providers use intense and aggressive linkages to community support systems, with continued oversight about how the consumer and the group interconnect (White & Kurtz, 2006).

For both mental health and addiction, recovery goes beyond "the elimination of symptoms from an otherwise unchanged life; it is about regaining wholeness, connection to a community, and a purpose-filled life" (White & Davidson, 2006a, p. 23). Also, in both mental health and addiction treatment fields, recovery support specialists (peer helpers) have become intrinsic to service programs (White & Kurtz, 2006; White & Davidson, 2006a,b).

PEER HELPERS

Peer- and recovery-support specialists in the fields of both mental health and addictions will be getting training and certification as the recovery models evolve. They find jobs in mental health and alcoholism and other drug treatment programs, where they facilitate group sessions, help consumers to access community resources, and make hospital visits. Their training incorporates the peer-support specialist's own recovery experience, which is a requirement for the position, as a means of inspiring hope in those they serve and also providing a positive role model. White and Kurtz (2006) listed functions of the recovery-support specialist in addictions as including the following: outreach worker, motivator, ally and confidant, truth teller, role model and mentor, planner, problem solver, resource broker, companion, advocate, educator, community organizer, lifestyle coach, and friend.

Likewise, peer-support specialists in mental health programs are nonprofessional peers who have experienced mental illness, have noticeably recovered, and have credibility with consumers experiencing symptoms and seeking service. Their role is to help the primary consumers to engage and continue services. This might include advocating for services, reminding them of and accompanying them to appointments, helping with practical tasks (such as furnishing an apartment, grocery shopping, opening bank accounts, using public transportation, etc.). They are not clinicians, but rather they are facilitators, advocates, and members of support systems.

Very often, peer helpers in mental health and addictions come from the ranks of mutual-help groups, where their own recovery has grown with the assistance provided by the group and the community of survivors that surrounds them.

In addiction services, the availability of recovering twelve-step group members involved in the treatment program has existed since the early days of the Minnesota Model. In mental health services, peer helper roles in the treatment agency are more recent. The literature on recovery in both mental health and addictions services fields reveals both similarities and differences. Table 2.2 contrasts key recovery approaches in the two service sectors. The goals and methods listed are general and not intended to catalog all the many activities that go into setting individual goals or interventions; they rather highlight the global outcomes and most representative methods in the recovery treatment literature, especially that of Joseph Walsh (2013) and William L. White (2005, 2008).

The concept of a transcendent recovery is listed as both a mental health and an addiction goal. It refers to the idea that some people "following the experience of addiction or mental illness, get 'better than well,' not in spite of the illness but because of the experiences and insight that emerged within their recovery processes" (White, Boyle, & Loveland, 2007, p. 236). This may be unrealistic for many people but can be a powerful goal for which to strive. I know this happens for people who give up a life of addiction and find a new life within the self-help community.

TABLE 2.2
COMPARISON OF MENTAL HEALTH AND ADDICTION RECOVERY APPROACHES

	Mental Health Recovery Approach	Addiction Recovery Approach
Goals/outcomes	Symptom accommodation Global health and development Responsibility and control of one's life Possessing recovery capital Transcendent recovery	Long-term recovery management (abstinence and sober living) A purpose-filled life Possessing recovery capital Transcendent recovery
Practice methods	Coping skills enhancement Psycho-education Peer support Transitional employment and housing Medication support and education Linking to community resources Long-term support	Recovery checkups Recovery coaching Stage-appropriate recovery education Linkages to recovering community Community resource development (supported work and housing) Long-term support

RECOVERY GROUPS

The goals listed for both sectors in table 2.2 are very similar. The methods comparison, however, points to a conspicuous difference between the two service sectors. A major focus in the addiction approach is linkage to communities of recovery, which in essence is linkage to local secular, spiritual, or religious mutual-aid groups and other recovery-support institutions. In the mental health sector, although peer helpers are included, linkage to community groups is less dominant in the literature. This should change according to a national estimate of mental health mutual-support groups; the authors reported existence of more than 1 million members in 3,315 mental health mutual-help groups in 2002 (Goldstrom et al., 2006).

Recovery groups can be a major source of peer support for people coping with mental illness or substance addictions. These groups in many cases affiliate with nationwide or international associations. In others, they may be local gatherings of people who meet in a mental health agency or consumer-run clubhouse. Some of the groups may be led by a professional, others by recovering peers. Modern recovery groups have been around since the mid-1930s in the United States and have spread to other countries around the world. They have been the hallmark of addiction recovery for the past half-century and a major, if not the only, source of extended support for addicts following treatment.

In the mental health field, one of the first recovery groups, WANA, initiated the founding of Fountain House in 1948. When John Beard took the helm of Fountain House in 1955, he introduced activity group therapy, a task-group intervention that became the model for clubhouse programs throughout the country (Doyle et al., 2013). Mental health self-help groups in the 1970s were of two basic types, the inner-focused individual-reform groups such as Recovery, Inc., and outer-focused social-reform groups such as the National Mental Health Consumers Association (Emerick, 1991). The outer-focused groups were more radical associations that rallied against the mental health establishment and decried psychiatric medications and psychiatric institutions. In the addictions arena, there has been a similar growth, from groups focusing on the intrapersonal and interpersonal dimensions of addiction recovery to groups advocating prorecovery social policies and programs and creation of recovery-friendly community environments. All of these varied groups contributed to the evolving recovery movement in the United States.

CONCLUSION

The modern recovery movement remains in a beginning stage, but it has had impact on federal behavioral health policy. In 2003, the final report of the President's New

Freedom Commission on Mental Health called for recovery to be the "common, recognized outcome of mental health services" (SAMHSA, 2003), and the Office of National Drug Control Policy stated in its 2012 ONDCP Recovery Update that the key to reducing American's drug problem is greater support for and partnership with the millions of citizens who are in long-term recovery from addiction (retrieved from http://www.whitehouse.gov/ondcp/recovery). (Chapter 10 will address the advocacy movement in more detail.)

Chapter 3 will introduce the kinds of groups most likely to serve as recovery groups: self-help mutual-aid and support groups. It will review the self-help ethos, differentiate the four types of groups that promote mental health and recovery, and describe how and when to use each model.

REFERENCES

Anderson, D. L., McGovern, J. P., & DuPont, R. L. (1999). The origins of the Minnesota Model of addiction treatment: A first person account. *Journal of Addictive Disease, 18*(1), 107–114.

Anderson, S. B. (1998). *We are not alone: Fountain House and development of clubhouse culture.* New York, NY: Fountain House.

Borkman, T. (2013). Special issue of Fountain House mental health clubhouses as hybrid self-help organizations. *International Journal of Self-Help and Self-Care, 7*(1), 1–6.

Chamberlin, J. (1978). *On our own: Patient-controlled alternatives to the mental health system.* New York, NY: McGraw-Hill.

Corrigan, P. W., & Ralph, R. O. (2005). Introduction: Recovery as consumer vision and research paradigm. In R. O. Ralph & P. W. Corrigan (Eds.), *Recovery in mental illness: Broadening our understanding of wellness* (pp. 3–17). Washington, DC: American Psychological Association.

Davidson, L., Tondora, J., Lawless, M. S., O'Connell, M. J., & Rowe, M. (2009). *A practical guide to recovery-oriented practice: Tools for transforming mental health care.* New York, NY: Oxford University Press.

Deegan, P. E. (2005). Recovery as a journey of the heart. In L. Davidson, C. Harding, & L. Spaniol (Eds.), *Recovery from severe mental illnesses: Research evidence and implications* (pp. 57–68). Boston, MA: Center for Psychiatric Rehabilitation, Boston University.

Doidge, N. (2007). *The brain that changes itself: Stories of personal triumph from the frontiers of brain science.* New York, NY: Penguin.

Doyle, A., Lanoil, J., & Dudek, K. (2013). *Fountain House: Creating community in mental health practice.* New York, NY: Columbia University Press.

Emerick, R. E. (1991). The politics of psychiatric self-help: Political factions, interactional support, and group longevity in a social movement. *Social Science and Medicine, 32*(10), 1121–1128.

Goldstrom, I. D., Campbell, J., Rogers, J. A., Lambert, D. B., Blacklow, B., Henderson, M. J., & Manderscheid, R. W. (2006). National estimates for mental health mutual support groups, self-help organizations, and consumer-operated services. *Administration and Policy in Mental Health and Mental Health Services Research, 33*(1), 92–103.

Granfield, R., & Cloud, W. (1999). *Coming clean: Overcoming addiction without treatment.* New York, NY: New York University Press.

Grohol, J. (2011). Mental illness is not simply a brain disease. Retrieved from http://psychcentral.com/blog/archives/2011/07/24/mental-illness-is-not-simply-a-brain-disease

Humphreys, K. (2004). *Circles of recovery: Self-help organizations for addictions.* Cambridge, UK: Cambridge University Press.

Jelinek, E. M. (1960). *The disease concept of alcoholism.* New Haven, CT: College and University Press.

Kalivas, P. W., & Volkow, N. C. (2005). The neural basis of addiction: A pathology of motivation and choice. *American Journal of Psychiatry, 162*(8), 1403–1413.

Karlsson, M. (2013). Introduction to mental health clubhouses: How the Fountain House clubhouse became an international model. *International Journal of Self-Help and Self-Care, 7*(1), 7–18.

Kurtz, L. F. (1984). Ideological differences between professionals and A.A. members. *Alcoholism Treatment Quarterly, 1*(2), 73–86.

Office of National Drug Control Policy. (n.d). Recovery (retrieved from http://www.whitehouse.gov/ondcp/recovery).

SAMHSA. (2003). *New Freedom Commission on Mental Health, achieving the promise: Transforming mental health care in America.* Final report. (DHHS Publication No. SMA-03-3832, Rockville, MD.) Available at www.mentalhealthcommission.gov

Spicer, J. (1993). *The Minnesota Model: The evolution of the multidisciplinary approach to addiction recovery.* Center City, MN: Hazelden.

Stanhope, V., & Solomon, P. (2013). Recovery-oriented services. In V. L. Vandiver (Ed.), *Best practices in community mental health* (pp. 185–198). Chicago, IL: Lyceum.

Walsh, J. (2013). *The recovery philosophy and direct social work practice.* Chicago, IL: Lyceum.

White, W., & Davidson, L. (2006a). System transformation. Recovery: The bridge to integration? (Part 1). *Behavioral Healthcare, 26*(11), 22–25.

White, W., & Davidson, L. (2006b). System transformation. Recovery: The bridge to integration? (Part 2). *Behavioral Healthcare, 26*(12), 24–26.

White, W., & Kurtz, E. (2006). Building relationships between treatment organizations and local communities of recovery. In *Linking addiction treatment and communities of recovery: A primer for addiction counselors and recovery coaches* (pp. 23–34). Pittsburgh, PA: IRETA.

White, W. L. (2005). Recovery: Its history and renaissance as an organizing construct concerning alcohol and other drug problems. *Alcoholism Treatment Quarterly, 23*(1), 3–15.

White, W. L. (2008). *Recovery management and recovery oriented systems of care: Scientific rationale and promising practices.* Pittsburgh, PA: IRETA.

White, W. L., Boyle, M., & Loveland, D. (2007). Recovery from addiction and mental illness: Shared and contrasting lessons. In R. O. Ralph & P. W. Corrigan (Eds.), *Recovery in mental illness: Broadening our understanding of wellness* (pp. 233–254). Washington, DC: American Psychological Association.

I alone can change my condition, but
I cannot do it alone.
RIESSMAN AND CARROLL (1995, p. 8)

3

HOW RECOVERY GROUPS DIFFER FROM OTHER KINDS OF GROUPS

PETER KROPOTKIN, A fifty-ish paunchy gentleman with a wild beard and rimless glasses, stayed for a while just before the turn of the twentieth century at Hull House in Chicago, where the social workers there described him as a "kindly scholar" (Addams, 1910/1960, p. 278). He was famous in Russian society for his advocacy of a nonviolent kind of revolutionary anarchism in which the state would be eliminated. In the United States, however, he is best known for his work on mutual aid. Although appreciative of Darwin's theory of evolution, he disagreed that the fittest survive through struggle and competition. A naturalist, Kropotkin concluded that cooperation, not competition, was the driving force behind the survival of a species, whether it was human, animal, or insect. In the introduction to his book, *Mutual Aid: A Factor of Evolution*, Kropotkin wrote: "I saw Mutual Aid and Mutual Support carried on to an extent which made me suspect in it a feature of the greatest importance for the maintenance of life, the preservation of each species, and its further evolution" (Kropotkin, 1902/1955, p. ix). Perhaps nowhere in American life has Kropotkin's insight been more evident than in the field of alcohol recovery.

When we think of recovery groups, we usually think first of twelve-step groups because they are ubiquitous in our society. There are other self-help associations that are less well known and some that fall into a societal reform category that we may not think of as recovery groups at all. One of those is MindFreedom International. MindFreedom represents a coalition of grass-roots activist associations formed around a mission of winning human rights and alternatives for people with a mental illness diagnosis (Brown & Wituk, 2010). Affiliated with it are about one hundred grass-roots groups around the world. These activist reform groups meet the definition of self-help groups and represent an important segment of the mental health recovering community. It was these reform-oriented groups for former mental patients that inspired the recovery model within the mental health field. The majority of groups for people with mental health histories, however, are the more self-reform types such as Recovery International and fall into the category labeled "mental health mutual-support group" in recent literature (Goldstrom et al., 2005). This chapter examines the self-help ethos and the subtypes of groups that exist in and around the recovery landscape in America.

SELF-HELP ETHOS AND RECOVERY PHILOSOPHY

Frank Riessman's (1965) "helper therapy principle" and Thomasina Borkman's (1976) concept of experiential knowledge are perhaps the two most seminal ideas from the early self-help literature. Riessman's idea was that the person who helps others is helped the most. The helper gains by achieving self-esteem, self-control, and competence; he or she can achieve perspective on his or her own problems and rehearse a new way of being in the act of helping someone who shares the same problem. Experiential knowledge is that which is gained by going through an experience. It is oriented to the here and now. When peers who have had the same experience come together, they do not question the other's ability to understand, empathize, and accept them. The feeling of being understood and the open natural communication between those with similar experiences is a critical feature of both self-help and support groups.

Riessman and Carroll (1995) wrote that the strength of the self-help movement of the 1970s lay in the spirit and worldview embodied in the self-help ethos. Its ideal type, they said, embodies an anti-big, antibureaucratic dimension, that is, against hierarchy, against impersonality, and against a division of labor that emphasizes technical competence. Self-help, by contrast, is personal; member competence is based on experience or experiential knowledge. Self-help can be construed as a politically conservative concept when compared with political support for government assistance and professional help. Members of self-help organizations, however, do not see themselves as replacements for others forms of assistance. Self-help becomes a form of empowerment and an expression of the democratic values that are inherent in the recovery philosophy. The self-help ethos, according to Riessman and Carroll, destigmatizes mental illness and disability and opens the door for participation in one's own healthcare. Their words in the mid-1990s foreshadowed the recovery movement that was to come in the next century.

TYPES OF GROUPS

Self-help or support groups come in many forms. Finding the right one is difficult, because there are so many types. Most people are familiar with twelve-step groups, such as the original, Alcoholics Anonymous. AA spread worldwide, a phenomenal development of the 1930s, when the Great Depression was winding down and a world war was about to begin. World War II launched AA into its first growth spiral, as members spread around the world, carrying with them the newly printed book *Alcoholics Anonymous: How Many Thousands of Men and Women Have Recovered from Alcoholism*. AA goes about its work quietly, and most people are unaware of the spread and influence of its 116,000 groups in the United States. AA is independent of professionals and institutions and has its own program of recovery, which has been imitated by hundreds of other fellowships for chemical and process addictions. (A process addiction is a compulsive form of a behavior such as gambling, sex, or eating.) It is one of the original and most successful recovery groups in the world. This is one type of self-help association: independent, nonprofessional, and complex.

A different self-help recovery model arose in the 1930s when Abraham Low, a neuropsychiatrist, developed a method of recovery from mental illness that he called "will training." He taught this method to groups of his patients who had left the hospital and needed follow-up care to prevent relapse. Low originally planned his aftercare meetings to be a modified psychotherapy type of group led by him, but he was pressured by his colleagues at the time to forgo this plan because it contradicted acceptable psychiatric practice. Over time, his method (codified in his 1950 book, *Mental Health Through Will Training*) caught on with the original group members, who demonstrated that they could practice the method without the psychiatrist by reading his book and discussing practice of his method together in weekly meetings. Thus, the original therapy group was transformed into a self-help group and spread throughout the nation and parts of the world as Recovery, Inc. (now Recovery International).

These methods have spawned the myriad associations that form the basis of the recovery movement in the United States and the world. Recovery groups fall into roughly two categories: self-help groups and support groups. What follows differentiates the two and then distinguishes them further from two other familiar types of groups.

Self-Help and Support Groups

Self-help (or mutual-help) groups must be differentiated from support groups, which are neither psychotherapy nor self-help in the strictest sense of the words. Support groups often have professional or trained leaders, but they do not offer psychotherapy. Structurally, they are usually simpler, smaller, and attached to a formal organization such as a hospital, a church or a social agency. Here are formal definitions of the two types of groups, first published in my book *Self-Help and Support Groups: A Handbook for Practitioners*:

> A self-help group is a supportive, educational, usually change-oriented, group that addresses a single life problem or condition shared by all members. Its purpose may be personal or societal change or both achieved through the use of original principles[1] for dealing with the situation. Its leadership is indigenous to the group's members; participation and contributions are voluntary—it charges no fees. Professionals rarely have an active role in the group's activities, unless they participate as members. Group boundaries include all who qualify for membership by having a problem, a situation, or an identity in common with other members. Meetings are structured and task-oriented and use specific methods of help for the basic problem or condition. Local groups are usually relatively autonomous from their national headquarters.
>
> Support groups meet for the purpose of giving emotional support and information to persons with common problems. They are often facilitated by professionals and linked to a social agency or a larger, formal organization. Membership criteria often exclude individuals not served by the sponsoring organization. Behavioral and societal changes are subordinate to the goals of emotional support and education. Meetings are relatively unstructured, and the group's program is unlikely to espouse a unique method.[2] Support groups usually do not charge fees or collect dues. (Kurtz, 1997, pp. 4–5)

Psychotherapy and Task Groups

It's important to differentiate self-help and support groups from psychotherapy and task groups, because how one relates to, initiates, and facilitates them differ. In the past, people have confused some of the well-known self-help groups such as AA with psychotherapy groups, because twelve-step groups can be therapeutic. However, the two types of group are not in competition with each other. Twelve-step groups help people get over serious, life-threatening addictions and illnesses, so why are they not therapy? Researchers have tried to study AA efficacy as if it were therapy but found this to be an impossible task—like comparing surgery with physical therapy. In many such studies, however, researchers have found that people who follow up treatment with AA attendance do better at maintaining recovery over time, and

---

[1] My original word for this was "ideologies."

[2] Originally "ideology."

recent outcome studies have found AA to be effective on its own. Nevertheless, AA-type self-help is not therapy. And the many support groups in existence are not therapy groups.

Therapy groups are made up of people selected for inclusion by a group therapist; self-help groups such as AA have open boundaries, admitting anyone with the problem addressed by the group. In therapy groups, the therapist controls the interaction by introducing topics, prodding for revelations, and interpreting group dynamics so that members will have new insights about themselves. Neither self-help nor support groups prod for revelations, interpret dynamics, or expect insights to be manifest. Interaction in therapy groups often follows a particular method of change, such as cognitive-behavioral therapy. AA and other complex mutual-aid groups also espouse a method of transformation, such as working through twelve steps, but this is a method devised by the founders and carried forward through group literature, not steered by a group therapist. Support groups may result in personal change, but that is not their primary goal.

Another type of group is a task group, which comes together for the purpose of completing a particular mission. Some examples are committees, work groups, study groups, and writing groups. An example of a task group related to recovery movement history is the activity group therapy initiated at Fountain House in 1956 by John Beard (Doyle, Lanoil, & Dudek, 2013; see chapter 12 below). While task groups often are supportive and educational, thus sharing characteristics with support groups, they differ in emphasis. Members are there to achieve a more specific goal. A psycho-education group is an example of a supportive task group. In this type, members learn about their or a family member's diagnosis and ways of managing recovery. Substance abuse treatment programs have used this type of group for many years.

Task groups are often time-limited; the task must be completed by a prescribed date. Others, such as staff groups, are regularly scheduled and highly task-oriented, conform to an agenda, and are led by an authority figure. Another example is a writing group that is more like a support group. It is a small group that meets in a senior center, with a supportive leader who encourages the elderly participants to write whatever they want and read it aloud. Along the way, they discuss whatever comes to mind, which often has to do with struggles to maintain independence as they age. This illustrates why it is hard to classify a group. The writing group is a task group that also provides support.

Ideal Types

You may be wondering which definition fits a group you have in mind but finding that you are unable to pinpoint it. That's because the definitions above describe ideal types. An ideal type is a construct that perfectly fits the definition. Reality rarely perfectly fits a construct. A group may have more of the characteristics of type one, and thus, generalizations about that type would apply to it, but it may also be similar in ways to type two. For example, a local chapter of the National Alliance on Mental Illness (NAMI) may be small and informal and meet in a mental health center but also be connected to the national association, which has a particular set of principles, indigenous leadership, and open boundaries.

Usually, those who attend self-help groups seek some kind of internal change: stopping an addiction, growing spiritually, becoming even-tempered, lessening depression, improving interpersonal relationships. These groups resemble psychotherapy groups in this respect. Some, in NAMI, for example, concentrate on a societal change, that is, increasing services for family members and changing laws, while at the same time giving support to families and people with a mental illness diagnosis. Support groups, however, do not typically emphasize a need for change within members or in society.

This differentiating is important because the kind of group you want to form or the kind of group you may inherit as a leader tells you what you should and should not do with it and what kinds of skills you need to apply in your role of initiator, leader, or facilitator.

Choosing a Group Type

Table 3.1 shows a comparison of the four group forms discussed here and key characteristics of each. Consider how you would approach an assignment in which you were asked to develop a new group of each type.

Forming a self-help group would require that you first find out if there is a national association for the particular problem you want to address and then learn from that group how they would advise you to start a group. Usually, there is a prepared packet of materials to use for this purpose. For example, the Depression and Bipolar Support Alliance (http://www.dbsalliance.org) has a page of instructions on its website and a start-up guide that is sent to a new group facilitator after an application is submitted.

If you are a professional and intend to develop a group that will meet in an agency, you need to find a national association that allows professional leadership or avoid that choice in favor of a more informal, local group. If you want to help members change in some way and to use a therapeutic method in doing so, you may need to choose the psychotherapy model instead of the support group model. If member education about the problems they face is one of your goals, then the support group or task group model is most likely to fit with your plan. If you want to form a group

TABLE 3.1
CHARACTERISTICS OF FOUR TYPES OF GROUPS

	Self-Help	Support	Psychotherapy	Task
Size	Large	Small	Small	Usually small
Change-oriented	Yes	No	Yes	No
Professionally led	No	Varies	Yes	Varies
Diagnosis/problem	Same	Same	Can differ	Does not apply
Educational focus	Sometimes	Usually	Rarely	Depends on task
Advocacy orientation	Depends on group	Often	No	Depends on task
National affiliation	Usually	Often	No	Depends on task
Professional agency affiliation	Never	Often	Usually	Depends on task

to accomplish a task, such as producing a program newsletter, then the task group model would work best.

Despite these many differences, there are aspects of all groups that make them successful, one of which is having appropriate structure for the group's purpose. It will be your task as the facilitator or leader to keep the group alive for the people in it. One of the aims of this book is to help you do that.

CONCLUSION

Self-help, support, mutual aid, and *mutual help* are all terms used to define groups that serve people who have something in common that causes distress. Some writers categorize self-help as one type of group and mutual support as another (Goldstrom et al., 2005). I have chosen to use the terms interchangeably, because my reading of the literature on the two does not show a uniform pattern of definition. I think the term *support*, however, does most often mean the same thing as my definition. The terms *psychotherapy* and *task* are much more precise when used in connection to groups, but practitioners do not always get adequate training in group work, so that using the wrong facilitator approach is both likely and unforgivable at the same time.

The next chapter will introduce some of the major self-help associations for mental health and addictions. There are hundreds of such groups, so the chapter will not include them all but will familiarize the reader with the wide range of associations that exist for dealing with addictions and mental health conditions, both twelve-step and non-twelve-step varieties.

REFERENCES

AA World Services. (1939). *Alcoholics Anonymous: How many thousands of men and women have recovered from alcoholism.* New York: Author.

Addams, J. (1910/1960). *Twenty years at Hull-House.* New York: New American Library.

Borkman, T. (1976). Experiential knowledge: A new concept for the analysis of self-help groups. *Social Service Review, 50,* 445–456.

Brown, L. D. & Wituk, S. A. (2010). *Mental health self-help: Consumer and family initiatives.* New York, NY: Springer.

Doyle, A., Lanoil, J., & Dudek, K. (2013). *Fountain House: Creating community in mental health practice.* New York, NY: Columbia University Press.

Goldstrom, I. D., Campbell, J., Rogers, J. A., Lambert, D. B., Blacklow, B., Henderson, M. J., & Manderscheid, R. W. (2005). National estimates for mental health mutual support groups, self-help organizations, and consumer-operated services. *Administration and Policy in Mental Health and Mental Health Services Research, 33*(1), 92–103.

Kropotkin, P. (1902/1955). Mutual aid: A factor of evolution. Boston, MA: Porter Sargent.

Kurtz, L. F. (1997). *Self-help and support groups: A handbook for practitioners.* Thousand Oaks, CA: Sage.

Low, A. A. (1950). *Mental health through will training.* Chicago, IL: Christopher Publishing House.

Riessman, F. (1965). The "helper-therapy" principle. *Social Work, 10,* 27–32.

Riessman, F., & Carroll, D. (1995). *Redefining self-help: Policy and practice.* San Francisco, CA: Jossey-Bass.

In the kinship of common suffering, one
alcoholic had been talking to another.
KURTZ (1979, p. 8)

4

GROUPS FOR ADDICTION AND MENTAL HEALTH CONDITIONS

THE MODERN SELF-HELP movement began in 1934, when Bill Wilson sat in his kitchen with Ebby T., a drinking buddy, who had just found religion. The Oxford Group was Ebby's solution to the relentless thirst for alcohol that had wrecked his life. From that moment forward, Wilson (known as Bill W.), the cofounder of Alcoholics Anonymous, set into motion a fellowship that would change the lives of millions of people around the world. He had one more binge after that founding moment, for which he dried out in New York City's Towns Hospital, where he experienced the "great peace" of religious conversion (Kurtz, 1979, p. 20). This experience led him to recognize the power of simultaneous deflation and hope—the power of one alcoholic talking to another. He envisioned a chain reaction among alcoholics, each one carrying this message and these principles to the next. Bill W., Dr. Bob S., and other early adherents brought that vision to life.

In 1938, the fledgling group of alcoholics took their message of recovery to Rock land State Hospital in upstate New York to share their story with the "hopeless" inebriates in custodial care in the alcoholism building. A psychiatrist, Dr. Hiram Johnson, watched the group of former alcoholics share their recovery with the inebriates, the alcoholics holding out promise for a new life outside the hospital. Johnson took the idea of such a group to another building, where he helped to form a self-help group of mental patients. That group of "hopeless" mental patients called itself We Are Not Alone (WANA). The first WANA members, after their release from Rockland State, returned to recruit others. WANA settled in Manhattan and found a building for its social activities in 1943; the members called it a clubhouse (Anderson, 1998). WANA did not survive long, but the clubhouse did, and it became Fountain House, the beginning of another movement for people thought to be hopelessly lost to an incurable mental illness.

That WANA failed to succeed as a self-help fellowship is not surprising, because starting a movement is a difficult undertaking. That AA and Fountain House survived and spread around the world to millions of people is a modern-day miracle. AA's method and organization, its Twelve Steps and Twelve Traditions, the small grass-roots meetings, its bottom-up structure, and its focus on members sharing stories have spread to hundreds of other fellowships for many of life's problems. This chapter will provide a sampling of many of those associations and others that fit the definition of self-help for people with addictions and mental health conditions. Fountain House will be discussed in chapter 12.

A lengthier discussion of twelve-step programs can be found in chapter 10. The fellowships listed in this chapter are a selection and should not be seen as the sum total of all fellowships available for people with addiction or psychiatric problems. Many are left out, which may seem unfair, but there are so many self-help associations in the United States that listing them all would add many pages to this short book. A complete listing can be found on the website of the American Self-Help Group Clearinghouse (http://www.mentalhelp.net/selfhelp), and most of those mentioned here, plus others, are at http://www.facesandvoicesofrecovery.org.

What follows begins with twelve-step associations for addicts; next, it covers a selection of non-twelve-step groups for addicts; it continues to review some of the twelve-step fellowships for mental health concerns, followed by a listing of non-twelve-step groups for mental health concerns, and it ends with associations for families.

TWELVE-STEP GROUPS FOR ADDICTION

Alcoholics Anonymous is an international fellowship, founded in 1935, with more than 114,000 in-person and online groups worldwide and more than 2 million members (AA, 2013). Its members come together to share their experience, strength, and hope, with the purpose of staying sober and helping other alcoholics to achieve sobriety. AA's headquarters are in New York City; its website (http://www.aa.org) provides information on literature and media, meeting locations, archives, and history. AA's Twelve Steps and Twelve Traditions form the substance of its program of recovery and its genius at organization. Its program has been examined repeatedly by researchers of all kinds, including social scientists (Galanter & Kaskutas, 2008; Humphreys, 2004), who have investigated outcomes of participation, and historians, who have published volumes on its beginning, founders, and history (AA, 1957; AA, 1984; Kurtz, 1979; Pittman, 1988; Thomsen, 1975).

Narcotics Anonymous is an international fellowship, founded 1953, with more than 61,000 in-person groups in the United States and 129 other countries. The only requirement for membership is a desire to stop using drugs. Its national headquarters are in Van Nuys, California; its website (http://www.na.org) offers information on how to start meetings, literature, events, discussion boards, and other resources. When people have addictions to more than one substance, some select one fellowship, and others attend meetings of more than one. John's story (box 4.1) is a case in point.

Alcoholics Victorious is an international fellowship, founded in 1948, with headquarters in Kansas City, Missouri. It has 170 in-person groups and uses the twelve steps and its own Alcoholics Victorious Creed in meetings. Its website (http://alco holicsvictorious.org) states that it offers a safe environment for recovering people who recognize Jesus Christ as their "Higher Power" and is a public service of the Association of Gospel Rescue Missions. The site gives information on its history, literature, meetings, and philosophy of addiction.

Cocaine Anonymous is an international twelve-step fellowship, founded in 1982, with 2,000 weekly in-person meetings in the United States, Canada, and the United Kingdom. Its headquarters are in Los Angeles. Its website (http://www. ca.org) states: "Cocaine Anonymous is concerned solely with the personal recovery and continued sobriety of anyone who wants to stop using cocaine and all other mind-altering substances (including alcohol and other drugs) and to help others achieve the same."

Crystal Meth Anonymous is an international twelve-step program, founded in 2000, with 500 weekly meetings. Membership is open to anyone with a desire to stop using drugs. It is headquartered in Los Angeles. Its website (http://www.crys talmeth.org)provides details on meeting locations and literature and other information about the fellowship.

Heroin Anonymous is an international twelve-step fellowship, founded in 2004, with meetings in fifty states and headquarters in Phoenix. Its website (http://www. heroinanonymous.org) contains information on literature and meetings in the United States, Canada, South Africa, and the United Kingdom. The site offers assistance in starting new meetings.

Marijuana Anonymous is an international twelve-step fellowship, founded in 1989with meetings in thirty-nine states, nine foreign countries, and online. It is headquartered in Van Nuys, California. The only requirement for membership is a desire to stop using marijuana. The group's website (http://www.marijuana-anonymous. org) offers daily online meetings led by a volunteer, a chat room, and an online newsletter. The website also provides extensive information about the fellowship, its meetings, its literature, and its program of recovery.

BOX 4.1
JOHN'S STORY

Many years after my first drinking experience, long after I had joined AA, I reflected that maybe it had started then, when I was thirteen. But it never really got off the ground. At eighteen, I tried heroin for the first time and forgot all about the childhood flirtation with beer.

Heroin was like coming home, to a home I had never known. The world became completely acceptable—not filled with joy or excitement, except for that first rush, but peaceful, until it turned on me, and I found myself totally wrapped up in chasing the next high, day after day, then year after year.

I went into a therapeutic community (TC) at thirty-two and then became a counselor, not knowing that I didn't know anything about counseling. I went on to direct TC treatment programs; I became a workaholic. Twelve years later, I suddenly started drinking alcoholically. In retrospect, my life had no sense of fulfillment, and my family suffered. I was on my way to finding out my problem wasn't the drug, it was me. I was an alcoholic.

Working in the substance abuse field, I drank secretly for eight years, until I was close to losing everything I had worked for—family, work, and friends. My wife knew but was powerless over it, then my children started to realize I had become a drunk, and finally, I was cornered and given the choice of losing everything or going to AA. Believe it or not, it was a hard decision to make. The fear and shame and guilt were overwhelming, almost enough to give up my life rather than face myself. I had become suicidal, at least in contemplation. There was a tree on the parkway that riveted my attention every time I drove past it, but I never got up the courage to swerve the wheel toward it.

Finally, one day, my wife told me she didn't know what I wanted to do with the rest of my life, but she was going to go to Al-Anon. That struck terror in my heart, and the next day, I went to AA, hoping no one who knew me would find out.

That was more than a quarter-century ago, and I have learned so many things since then (and had to relearn many of them, several times over). I remember well the day my first sponsor suggested I share at least something at every meeting. "Share your strength, hope, and experience, tell them how you are doing today, and then shut up." He told me that when I introduced myself in an AA meeting by name and said I was an alcoholic, I told them everything important about me—the rest was superfluous. By exaggeration, he helped me accept myself as I was. A quarter-century later, I look back on a full and unfinished life and forward to opportunity but, most of all, to today. Life is good.

Methadone Anonymous Support is an international twelve-step fellowship founded in 1991 with meetings in most states and online. It is open to people with addictions who use methadone to maintain their recovery from use of opiates, alcohol, and other drugs. Its website (http://www.methadonesupport.org) directs visitors to meetings and to online chat rooms. The website also links to literature and online forums.

Nicotine Anonymous is an international twelve-step fellowship, founded in 1980, with in-person meetings in thirty-six states and thirty-five countries. It is a group of men and women helping one another to live lives free of nicotine: "The only requirement for membership is the desire to stop using nicotine" (http://www.nicotine-anonymous.org). Information is available in thirteen languages. Headquarters are in Huntington Beach, California.

NON-TWELVE-STEP GROUPS FOR ADDICTION

The Buddhist Recovery Network is an international association, founded in 2008, with groups in nineteen states and Australia, Canada, Thailand, Northern Ireland, and the United Kingdom. It is headquartered in Marylhurst, Oregon. Its website (http://www.buddhistrecovery.org) lists meetings, resources, and events. The Buddhist Recovery Network supports the use of Buddhist teachings, traditions, and practices to help people recover from the suffering caused by addictive behaviors. Open to people of all backgrounds and respectful of all recovery paths, the organization promotes mindfulness and meditation and is grounded in Buddhist principles of nonharming, compassion, and interdependence. It seeks to serve an international audience through teaching, training, treatment, research, publication, advocacy, and community-building initiatives.

Jewish Alcoholics, Chemically Dependent Persons, and Significant Others (JACS) was founded in 1978 and is headquartered in New York. It has fifty groups in nineteen states, Canada, Australia, Brazil, and Israel. Its website (http://www.jbfcs.org) explains its program and history and contains links to meeting locations. JACS assists the Jewish community in exploring recovery in a nurturing Jewish environment. It is a self-help/mutual-aid movement of recovering Jewish people empowering themselves, talking to their communities, and advocating for services on behalf of addicted Jews and their families.

Secular Organizations for Sobriety, founded in 1985, has 750 groups and online fellowship. It is headquartered in Hollywood, California. Its website (http://www.sossobriety.org) states: "SOS is an alternative recovery method for those alcoholics or drug addicts who are uncomfortable with the spiritual content of widely available

12-Step programs. SOS takes a reasonable, secular approach to recovery and maintains that sobriety is a separate issue from religion or spirituality. SOS credits the individual for achieving and maintaining his or her own sobriety, without reliance on any 'Higher Power.'"

LifeRing began in 2001 as an offshoot of SOS. It has 115 in-person groups, online activity in a chat room, and a discussion forum. It is headquartered in Oakland, California. Its website (http://lifering.org) offers information on the program, links to local meetings, a newsletter, and a bookstore. LifeRing is not affiliated with any other organization and is independent financially, legally, and organizationally. LifeRing meetings are started and led by peer volunteers called conveners.

SMART Recovery (Self-Management and Recovery Training), established in 1994, is headquartered in Mentor, Ohio, and sponsors 950 weekly, face-to-face groups and thirty online meetings. Its website (http://www.smartrecovery.org) describes it as "a self-empowering, science-based mutual support group for abstaining from any substance or activity addiction. It teaches tools organized under the 4-Point Program: (1) Building and Maintaining Motivation, (2) Coping With Urges, (3) Managing Thoughts, Feelings, and Behaviors and (4) Living a Balanced Life." The site has links to national and international meeting locations, leadership manuals, and online resources for members and their families. SMART Recovery trains its own group facilitators in an eight-week online course.

Women for Sobriety, founded in 1976 and headquartered in Quakertown, Pennsylvania, has 200 in-person and online groups. It is an organization dedicated to helping women overcome alcoholism and other addictions. The WFS "New Life" program grew out of one woman's search for sobriety. Its website (http://www.womenforsobriety.org) contains meeting information, instructions for group moderators, and an online store. Kaskutas (1989) conducted a survey of WFS members. Goals of membership included abstinence, improved self-esteem, and spiritual and emotional growth. About a third of the respondents currently attended AA in addition to WFS.

TWELVE-STEP GROUPS FOR MENTAL HEALTH CONDITIONS

Some of the groups described here include families of people with addictions, in addition to mental health or behavioral problems, and one is for people with dual problems of alcohol and psychiatric disability.

Depressed Anonymous is a twelve-step fellowship providing groups or circles of support for persons who are depressed. It seeks to inform and educate the public about the signs and symptoms of depression and advises people on where they can go to seek help and to establish self-help programs in their own communities. It is headquartered in Louisville, Kentucky, and has groups in thirteen states and six countries outside the United States. An online discussion group is offered on its website (http://www.depressedanon.com).

Emotions Anonymous is an international fellowship, founded in 1971, with 1,000 chapters. It is headquartered in St. Paul, Minnesota. Its website (http://www.emotionsanonymous.org) gives information on the locations of meetings, literature, and online discussions. The site states: "EA is a 12-Step fellowship of people who come together for the purpose of working toward recovery from emotional difficulties. EA is most suitable for people who want to use the 12 steps for emotional concerns not limited by diagnosis and for those who already attend AA or NA, but is open to anyone who feels a need for recovery from emotional conditions."

Dual Recovery Anonymous is a nonprofessional, independent, twelve-step-based self-help association for people with a dual diagnosis of chemical dependency and emotional or psychiatric illnesses (see chapter 10). It was founded in 1989 and has 880 in-person meetings. Its headquarters are in Prairie Village, Kansas. Its website (http://www.draonline.org) explains its program and lists meeting locations.

NON-TWELVE-STEP GROUPS FOR MENTAL HEALTH CONDITIONS

Non-twelve-step self-help, mutual-aid groups for mental health conditions include many very old organizations such as Recovery International (1937) and newer ones such as Bipolar World (1998), an online-only group. As with twelve-step fellowships, there are many groups for people with psychiatric diagnoses that will not be listed here. Complete listings can be found at http://www.mentalhelp.net/selfhelp.

The Depression and Bipolar Support Alliance was founded in Chicago in 1986 as the Manic Depressive and Depressive Association and then became the National Depressive and Manic Depressive Association before its recent name change. DBSA has 1,000 groups, including 700 support groups and 300 chapters; it offers online peer support. Its website (http://www.dbsalliance.org) contains a meeting locator, news, access to online groups, literature, and links to other sites of interest. The website states: "The Depression and Bipolar Support Alliance (DBSA) is the leading peer-directed national organization focusing on the two most prevalent mental health conditions, depression and bipolar disorder, which affect more than 21 million Americans, account for 90% of the nation's suicides every year, and cost $23 billion in lost workdays and other workplace losses."

GROW is an international association with 650 groups in the United States, Australia, New Zealand, Ireland, and other countries. GROW's American headquarters are in Champaign-Urbana, Illinois (http://www.growinamerica.org). GROW International was originally organized in Australia. GROW in America is fully developed in Illinois and New Jersey, with some groups in Rhode Island. People come to GROW with diverse problems in living, such as mental health, emotional troubles, or difficulty coping with grief, loneliness, anxiety, or stress. GROW offers leadership training and consultation to develop new groups. This association has been studied intensely in the United States and in Australia (Rappaport et al., 1985; Finn, Bishop & Sparrow, 2007).

Recovery International (see chapter 10) is headquartered in Chicago, where it began in 1937. It has more than 600 in-person groups and offers groups online. It describes itself as "A community mental health mutual aid group that offers a self-help method of will training: a system of techniques for controlling temperamental behavior and changing attitudes toward nervous symptoms, anxiety, depression, anger and fears." Its website (http://www.lowselfhelpsystems.org) provides help with starting new groups, a meeting locator, and results of evaluations of its cognitive/behavioral program. Recovery International has been the subject of numerous research activities, the most recent being an evaluation by Susan Pickett, which is available on the Recovery International website (Pickett, Phillips, & Kraus, 2011).

MindFreedom International is a nonprofit organization that unites 100 sponsor and affiliate grass-roots groups with thousands of individual members to win human rights and alternatives for people labeled with psychiatric disabilities. Its website (http://www.mindfreedom.org) states that its goals are to "win human rights campaigns in mental health, challenge abuse by the psychiatric drug industry, support the self-determination of psychiatric survivors and mental health consumers, promote safe, humane and effective options in mental health." MindFreedom is physically based in Eugene, Oregon; however, its activities occur in other locations with its affiliated grass-roots groups.

The National Alliance on Mental Illness (see chapter 11) is an advocacy association that also sponsors support groups for people who have psychiatric disabilities and their families. Its headquarters are in Arlington, Virginia. Its website (http://www.nami.org) states that it is "the nation's largest grassroots mental health organization dedicated to building better lives for the millions of Americans affected by mental illness. NAMI advocates for access to services, treatment, supports and research and is steadfast in its commitment to raise awareness and build a community for hope for all of those in need." Schizophrenics Anonymous (see chapter 10) is a program of the larger Schizophrenia and Related Disorders Alliance of America and is a self-help association for persons who have schizophrenia or schizophrenia-related illnesses. In spite of the "Anonymous" in its name, SA is not a twelve-step fellowship. It was founded in the Detroit area in July 1985. There are currently more than 150 groups meeting throughout thirty-one states and in Australia, Brazil, Canada, Mexico, France, India, and Venezuela. The SA website is at http://www.sardaa.org/schizophrenics-anonymous.

GROUPS FOR FAMILIES AND FRIENDS

Al-Anon Family Groups is an international twelve-step fellowship, founded in 1955, the first family-and-friend fellowship to be established (see chapter 10). There are more than 24,000 in-person groups in 115 countries. Membership includes men, women, and children whose lives have been affected by a family member's or friend's drinking. Al-Anon sponsors a subfellowship for the children of alcoholics called Alateen. Al-Anon's headquarters is in Virginia Beach, Virginia, and its website is at http://www.al-anon.alateen.org. Al-Anon's focus is on the member, not the drinking alcoholic. All family members, children, spouses, parents, friends, employers, and employees are welcome.

Nar-Anon Family Groups is an international fellowship for those affected by someone else's drug addiction, which includes alcohol. Its headquarters are in Torrance, California, and its website is at http://www.nar-anon.org. As a twelve-step program, Nar-Anon offers help by sharing experience, strength, and hope among participants. The only requirement for membership is addiction in a relative or friend.

Co-Anon Family Groups is international, with groups in thirteen states, Canada, and the United Kingdom. Co-Anon is a twelve-step fellowship of men and women who are husbands, wives, parents, relatives, or close friends of someone who is dependent on cocaine. Co-Anon's "EMeeting" has more than 300 members on five continents and functions as an e-mail group. Co-Anon literature can be ordered through its website (http://www.co-anon.org). It is headquartered in Tucson, Arizona.

Families Anonymous is an international fellowship with 500 in-person groups and online discussions. It is headquartered in Culver City, California. Its website (https://www.familiesanonymous.org) gives information on meeting locations, literature and other materials, the program, and upcoming events. FA is a twelve-step fellowship for families and friends who have known a feeling of desperation concerning the destructive behavior of someone very near to them, whether caused by drugs, alcohol, or related behavioral problems.

The family fellowships described here are open to members without regard to whether the family member with an addiction has entered a fellowship or begun recovery.

CONCLUSION

Chapter 10 will discuss Al-Anon Family Groups, Recovery International, Schizophrenics Anonymous, and Dual Recovery Anonymous in more detail than this chapter has done. Chapter 11 will describe some of the political and advocacy activities of groups, and chapter 13 will describe online groups. Next, though, chapter 5 will address ways in which mental health and addiction treatment personnel can work cooperatively with independent self-help associations like those listed above. It will emphasize the importance of the linking act in which the professional helps someone become attached to a self-help community of groups and members.

REFERENCES

AA. (1957). *Alcoholics Anonymous comes of age*. New York, NY: AA Publishing.

AA. (1984). *Pass it on: The story of Bill Wilson and how the A.A. message reached the world.* New York, NY: AA World Services.

AA. (2013). *Estimates of groups and members*. Service material. New York: AA World Services. Retrieved from www.aa.org

Anderson, S. B. (1998). *We Are Not Alone: Fountain House and the development of clubhouse culture.* New York: Fountain House.

Finn, L., Bishop, B., & Sparrow, N. (2007). Mutual help groups: An important gateway to well-being and mental health. *Australian Health Review, 31*, 246–255.

Galanter, M., & Kaskutas, L. A. (2008). *Research on Alcoholics Anonymous and spirituality in addiction recovery.* New York, NY: Springer.

Humphreys, K. (2004). *Circles of recovery: Self-help organizations for addictions.* New York, NY: Cambridge University Press.

Kaskutas, L. A. (1989). Women for Sobriety: A qualitative analysis. *Contemporary Drug Problems, 16*(2), 177–200.

Kurtz, E. (1979). *Not-God: A history of Alcoholics Anonymous.* Center City, MN: Hazelden.

Pickett, S., Phillips, H., & Kraus, D. (2011). *Recovery International group meeting evaluation: Final report.* Available at http://www.lowselfhelpsystems.org/documents/ri_final_report_3.1.11.pdf

Pittman, B. (1988). *AA: The way it began*. Seattle, WA: Glen Abbey Books.

Rappaport, J., Seidman, E., Toro, P., McFadden, L., Reischl, T., Roberts, L., et al. (1985). Collaborative research with a mutual help organization. *Social Policy, 15*, 12–24.

Thomsen, R. (1975). *Bill W.* New York, NY: Harper & Row.

2

[H]e was sure there was hope somehow
for him and that this doctor with his
hand on his shoulder was encouraging
him to do his part.
RAU AND RAU (1971, p. 107)

5

CONNECTING WITH INDEPENDENT SELF-HELP RECOVERY GROUPS

ABRAHAM LOW, THE Chicago neuropsychiatrist mentioned in chapter 3, believed that Freud's ideas about the origins and cure of mental illness could not possibly be right. He developed unique, common-sense methods of aftercare for his patients from both his lifelong study of language and his experience in helping people who had been hospitalized for mental illness. Today, Recovery International's method is known as cognitive-behavioral training, which Low called "will training"; he taught it to his individual patients and to people he met in aftercare groups (Low, 1950). He did not intend to start a self-help organization; he thought of his groups as simplified therapy groups for recovering patients led by psychiatrists. Fortunately, perhaps, he could never find another psychiatrist willing to use his method. Through a series of missed opportunities and outright condemnation by the professional medical establishment, Recovery, Inc. never caught on with formal mental health practitioners, but it did catch on with its members, and this led to the first of the modern-day self-help associations for mental health conditions in the world (Boyer, unpublished).

Low had encouraged his former patients to organize an advocacy association for the purpose of fighting stigma and changing commitment laws (Low, 1943). They had incorporated their group as Recovery, Inc., in 1937 for that purpose. The advocacy groups made little progress; the legal change they pushed for was passed in the Illinois legislature but vetoed by the governor. With advocacy efforts a failure, the groups evolved into small self-help therapy groups. When Low announced the end of his group therapy practice, his former patients refused to break up and continued holding meetings throughout Cook County. Low maintained contact with the Chicago organization for the rest of his life; he wrote a book on will training for members, recorded lectures for groups to play in meetings, and continued to see members privately until his death in 1954 (Rau and Rau, 1971). Low referred to his method and the groups as "self-help." This was likely the first use of the term as applied to member-led groups.

FOUNDERS

Although Low had a traumatic childhood, he did not found his groups as an acknowledged fellow sufferer. His intended mission was to bring his method to state hospitals, where the majority of people with psychiatric problems suffered, but he met with resistance from administrators and officials at every turn. He failed in those efforts, the last in Michigan just before his death. It took Low a long time to realize that a group such as his could meet without him or some other psychiatrist. Ultimately, he found that average nonprofessionals were more capable and willing than the psychiatrists of the day, who could not give up the outdated theories they held. More than fifty years would pass before the psychiatric profession would open its collective mind to groups such as Recovery International (its later name).

Father Con Keogh was a fellow sufferer who dedicated the last years of his life to mutual help for the mentally ill (Keogh, 1979, pp. 10–11). In 1953, the Catholic priest, who taught at a seminary in Australia, experienced a mental breakdown. He was hospitalized and given electroconvulsive treatments, which left him shattered. He looked for a group for people like himself but could find only AA. He credited the AA fellowship as the source of his eventual recovery. From that point until he died in 2011, Keogh devoted his life to the fellowship he founded, which he called GROW. He borrowed much of his program from AA's twelve-step model and would later add some of Recovery International's will training to GROW's program. Nevertheless, GROW has a distinct worldview and method of operation that have allowed it to spread from Australia to the United States and other countries (Salem, Seidman, & Rappaport, 1988). Although Keogh was a clergyman, he was also a former mental patient, which gave him a perspective that nonsufferers did not have.

AA, founded by Bill Wilson and Dr. Bob Smith, is another self-help fellowship that owes its existence to two fellow sufferers. In addition to Wilson and Smith, others contributed to the success and development of the AA program. One Catholic clergyman, Father Edward Dowling in St. Louis, supported both AA and Recovery, Inc., by helping to start groups and counseling members (Rau & Rau, 1971). The founders' stories, especially Wilson's, demonstrate the boundless dedication it took to mount a successful movement for recovering people. Both of the founders devoted the rest of their lives to the AA fellowship; for Wilson, this stretched thirty-four years to his death in 1971.

When you consider the long years of effort these founders gave to the task, it's easy to see why hundreds of mutual-help groups have adopted the twelve-step program rather than go through the work of fashioning a new one. But developing an entirely new program is possible, as shown by people who established more recent associations. These include Jean Kirkpatrick, founder of Women for Sobriety; Alan Marlatt, cofounder of Buddhist Recovery Network; and James Christopher, founder of Secular Organization for Sobriety. You can dedicate your life to beginning a self-help fellowship like the people just discussed, or you can keep it simple by starting a local chapter of a fellowship already in existence.

STARTING A LOCAL CHAPTER

If you want to begin a local chapter of a national self-help association, most make it easy. Go to the group's website and look for directions. Some, like Recovery International, ask that you call them; others tell you to e-mail them for assistance. Most of the groups—Emotions Anonymous, for example—offer a starter packet that includes literature, instructions on how meetings work, and a suggested format for meetings. Some ask for registration or a charter with the parent organization.

I used to say that a true self-help association did not allow for professional facilitators, but there are a few exceptions. GROW trains professionals as sponsors only; however, professionals have served as group leaders during its development period in Illinois (Toro et al., 1988). Schizophrenics Anonymous also recruited professional group leaders during a development period in Michigan (Salem, Reischl, & Randall, 2008). Smart Recovery uses volunteer professional and nonprofessional leaders; the organization provides thirty hours of facilitator training online, for which there is a monetary fee.

Once you have a starter packet from a self-help association, you can use it to guide the development of your own materials for a core group of members. You may take the leader role in the beginning, or you may assist your core membership to assume group leadership. Assuming that your group members have already identified the national self-help association with which they wish to ally themselves, the starter packet will contain information on the program, advice for developing an agenda for meetings, and group literature to be either sold or given to members. Literature usually is for sale on organization websites and can be purchased in bulk to resell. The local chapter must have the funds to purchase the initial order. If you are the staff person who is organizing the group, you must decide how to frame your role as a helper and consultant and not the group leader. Will you attend meetings, or will you stay on the sidelines as a consultant? If the group succeeds, you will be more involved in the beginning than you will be later.

The newly formed group may need help publicizing itself so that it will gain credibility in the community. You will have to decide whether the group will meet at the agency or in the community; if the latter, you may need to help find a place to meet, such as a church basement or a hospital meeting room. Twelve-step groups pay rent for the places they meet, using contributions they receive from participants. You should be prepared to offer advice about group facilitation to the leaders, although much of what they need to know can be learned by observing meetings of other self-help groups in the community. Such groups typically meet in a circle, with members taking turns sharing within the group. Many discourage crosstalk in order to make time for everyone to have a say. Groups often toss out a theme for each meeting; this is one way to discourage an emphasis on problems and complaints and to encourage solutions and methods of applying the program philosophy and teachings. In chapter 6, I will discuss starting and facilitating meetings in more depth.

When it comes to recovery-oriented practice, the founding and starting of community recovery groups is arguably much less important than linking people to the groups. Outcome research has established the importance of self-help involvement after treatment for addictions, and the recovery model of care focuses on the need for attention to linking people to a group network (Humphreys, 2004; White & Kurtz, 2006).

LINKING PEOPLE WITH SELF-HELP

Treatment staff members must "strengthen their relationships with diverse communities of recovery and enhance and individualize their strategies for linking clients" to them (White & Kurtz, 2006, p. 18). Recovery methods in both substance abuse and mental health sectors involve helping people connect with others in self-help/support groups, clubhouses, or other places where they can find acceptance and form nondrinking, nonusing social relationships. For substance abusers, the using community is out there waiting to lure them back. Something intensely persuasive must counter that temptation.

Although the research shows that connecting people to self-help and support group communities leads to better outcomes (Timko & DeBenedetti, 2007), formal treatment organizations have been deficient in their ability to link people with communities of recovery (Davidson, Tondora, Lawless, O'Connell, & Rowe, 2009;

Powell & Perron, 2010; White & Kurtz, 2006). Peer helpers, on the other hand, often guide newly recovering people to resources, assist them in finding community groups, and provide ongoing support and friendship. Being part of a self-help group offers members a chance to help others, achieve a sense of mattering, and realize identity transformation, all of which support sobriety and self-acceptance (Conrad-Garrisi & Pernice-Duca, 2013; Finn, Bishop, & Sparrow, 2009; Mandiberg & Edwards, 2013). This highlights the importance of the twelfth step, carrying the message and helping others. The twelfth step came from AA's very beginning, when Ebby T. visited Bill W. to bring him hope for recovery in the Oxford Group.

When I was a community mental health practitioner, I saw some people whose abuse of substances put them into the hospital over and over again. They would complete an inpatient stay of a few weeks, go home or stay in a halfway house for a while, look for work, go to meetings of AA, find a place to live, and sometimes find a job. Soon after they began work or began living independently, they would get drunk, and the whole multistage scenario would begin over again. One person I remember well had the distinction of having the most inpatient admissions of all time. "Revolving-door" alcoholics become extreme examples of people who need extended recovery management. They have exhausted their resources and are unable to tolerate the slightest stress without using their drug of choice, and once they use, recovery stalls. Brief inpatient stays give them detox from the drug and a few weeks of sobriety before they come out and try drinking or drugging again.

Research literature reports that the majority of those who complete addiction treatment resume alcohol or drug abuse within a year (White & Kurtz, 2006). Those who obtain help, such as attendance at AA or NA, are more likely to remain abstinent from alcohol or free of drugs (Kaskutas, 2009; Moos & Moos, 2006). However, only one in five clients receives professionally directed postdischarge continuing care. Kelly and Moos (2003) followed a large sample of men (n = 2,778) after treatment and found that 40 percent of their subjects dropped out of AA by the end of one year following discharge from care. The men were less likely to drop out, they found, if they had initiated AA contact during treatment. They concluded that high-risk consumers would be at lower risk if they received more supportive care during treatment than what had been offered to them. The presence on staff of recovery coaches who can facilitate early involvement in AA or other recovery groups should increase their group participation after treatment.

In another study, researchers compared those who received intensive discharge planning with those who received only the standard referral process and found that the more intensive methods were more effective (Timko & DeBenedetti, 2007). Intensive linking consisted of providing information on self-help meetings, reviewing group literature, addressing common concerns about participation, and introducing the patient to a member of AA or NA. Furthermore, the researchers asked patients in the intensive condition to keep a journal recording the meetings they attended and their thoughts about each meeting. They recruited self-help volunteers who were linked with patients needing AA or NA sponsors. Treatment staff monitored failures to follow through on referrals and made repeated efforts to connect former patients with groups and sponsors. People linked with twelve-step groups in the manner just described followed through with meeting attendance more than control subjects and got more involved in the groups in other ways, such as reading literature and providing service. Persons receiving the intensive intervention also used substances less frequently and were more likely to be abstinent.

For psychiatrically disabled persons who return to the community after treatment, the challenge is not so much about refraining from drug and alcohol misuse, although this is a concern, as it is about whether the persons find safe living conditions that they can afford, recreational and social opportunities, and employment. These needs typically fall to the case manager in a mental health service. Social policy experts Mechanic and Aiken (1989/2011) criticized public mental health care in 1989, pointing out that programs had to staff agencies with the lowest level of workers as a result of inadequate funding, with the case manager's role being lowest in rank, lowest in pay, and lowest in educational preparation. If case management is to be effective, they said, it must be embedded in a system that has the resources available to provide the full spectrum of service elements. These services include housing, social welfare benefits, medical evaluations, medication management, and vocational rehabilitation. Most of these services are also needed for returning substance abusers. In addition to the four services just mentioned, case managers are also those who will need to use the aggressive linking to the self-help communities referred to in box 5.1.

Some people with psychiatric disabilities can return to full functioning without obvious symptoms. Those in this fortunate segment of the affected population need only to receive the best medicine can offer them and can then return to a life unaltered by their period of illness. For many, however, this is not possible in the near term, and their life course can be damaged considerably when they have to stay in jail or be homeless for long periods. A study in 2010 found that 16 percent of the inmates in jails and prisons had a mental illness diagnosis (approximately 362,693 U.S. citizens) (Torrey, Kennard, Eslinger, Lamb, & Pavle, 2010). The National Alliance to End Homelessness (http://www.endhomelessness.org) reported that "on a given night in 2012, nearly 40% of the homeless population had serious mental illness or conditions related to chronic substance abuse" (approximately 257,226 U.S. citizens). Society must find a way to change these statistics. Linking to community

BOX 5.1
STEPS IN THE ASSERTIVE LINKING PROCESS

- Educating clients about the importance and potential benefits of posttreatment recovery support services.
- Soliciting clients' past experience with solo experiments in sobriety.
- Soliciting clients' past experience with and perceptions of recovery mutual-aid groups.
- Reviewing the menu of posttreatment recovery support options.
- Identifying important meeting characteristics.
- Using assertive rather than passive linking procedures, such as orienting clients regarding what to expect in the first meeting.
- Linking each client to a particular person from a list of volunteer guides to orient and guide the client into relationship with a local group and linking each client to a specific meeting for initial exposure.
- Demonstrating personal enthusiasm and optimism to clients about recovery-support participation.
- Resolving obstacles to participation, such as day care or transportation.
- Clarifying the role differences among counselor, recovery coach, and group sponsor to avoid confusion, conflicting loyalties, and manipulative attempts to evade responsibility by clients
- Monitoring and evaluating each client's initial and ongoing responses to the person or meeting via follow-up phone calls, e-mails, or visits.
- Providing support for continued contact or exploring alternatives in response to mismatches between person and group.
- Linking family members to support structures congruent with the recovery framework of a client, such as referring spouses and children to family groups when available.

From White and Kurtz (2006). Although this list is for recovery from addiction, most of the points also apply to mental health recovery.

recovery groups will not solve these problems, but it is a crucial aspect of follow-up care that must be addressed.

What is the linker role, and how can professionals, treatment staff, recovery coaches, and others become better at doing it? The process requires more than giving the person a list of groups at discharge and expecting that person to find a meeting place, attend a meeting, and keep going back. Traditional aftercare provides follow-up visits with a clinician who relies on verbal encouragement for participation in recovery groups following discharge (White & Kurtz, 2006). This is not enough, and referral is not the same as linking. According to White and Kurtz

(2006, p. 35), "linkage is a process that assures that the connection between an individual and the indigenous recovery support systems really happens." They recommend the linkage steps in box 5.1.

Linking practices in most substance abuse treatment facilities begin with having local groups meet in the facility, either as a regularly scheduled meeting for the community or as a group specifically intended to introduce new patients to AA, NA, or other self-help groups, such as Women for Sobriety. Follow-up strategies aim to hook treatment graduates into the social world of AA and other local twelve-step groups. Because of the density of twelve-step groups, they can and do become a community or social world (Smith, 2007). For example, an individual attends meetings, locates a job through the contacts he or she makes in the group, hangs out at the local Alano Club (a private club for recovering people), and finds a roommate with whom to share housing. In 270 communities throughout the United States, there are Oxford Houses that provide a place to live with other recovering people who adhere to the twelve-step program of AA or NA (see chapter 12). The Oxford House offers a more intense twelve-step experience than independent living and exists within the local social world of recovering people.

The recommendations in box 5.1 also apply to mental health self-help groups. The largest national associations for psychiatric rehabilitation are listed in chapter 4. Formal mental health agencies can support peer-operated services by hosting local, regional, and state group meetings and advocacy activities for people in recovery and their families, such as those of NAMI, Emotions Anonymous, Recovery International, Schizophrenics Anonymous, and GROW (Davidson et al., 2009).

My studies in the 1980s (Kurtz, 1984; Kurtz, 1985; Kurtz, Mann, & Chambon, 1987) found that 86 percent of substance abuse treatment directors and staff members linked consumers to AA and that a similar number, 84 percent, of mental health social workers referred or linked clients with AA and other self-help groups not directly related to mental illness. For the 1987 study, we selected a sample of mental health social workers whose agencies were located near existing mental health self-help groups (Recovery, Inc.; Emotions Anonymous; GROW; or the Manic Depressive and Depressive Association [MDDA]) and asked if they linked consumers with any of those groups. A much lower percentage (54 percent) linked to any of the mental health groups. Most (79 percent) reported that a lack of information was why they did not link clients to mental health groups. Recovery, Inc., was most familiar to the social workers (46 percent) but received fewer referrals (32 percent) than the MDDA, which was less familiar to the social workers (33 percent) but received 34 percent of the referrals. Emotions Anonymous and GROW received the fewest referrals (16 percent and 14 percent). It seemed mental health social workers were less familiar with and less likely to refer to groups that most fit the mental health needs of their consumers and whose programs were most similar to those of the social work agency. This fits with the theory that a formal agency would be less inclined to cooperate and link clients with an obvious competitor; however, it may have been that these groups with fewer affiliates than AA were just as they said, simply unfamiliar to the workers.

The mental health social workers reported that those they linked with the self-help groups did not follow through with the referrals (about one-fourth to one-third), that many of those who did follow through did not continue attendance, and that only about one-third appeared to receive help from the groups. When asked what kinds of linking activities the social workers thought were appropriate, referring was the activity most chosen (80 percent); consultation, speaking before a group, and attending meetings were other activities that received more than 50 percent of their choices. By referring, they meant that they told the client about the group and where it met. The activities least preferred were having group members volunteer at the agency (17 percent) and hiring group members to work in the agency (8 percent). Based on what we know today, these least-preferred methods are the ones most likely to be effective. These data from twenty-six years ago evidence attitudes that are inconsistent with attitudes needed to practice within today's recovery paradigm, which advocates peer helping.

PROFESSIONAL LEADERSHIP OF SELF-HELP GROUPS

To most of us, a *self-help* group is by definition one that helps itself without professional leadership. The term also connotes mutual help, suggesting that the members help one another in the groups and also between meetings. Two self-help associations for people with mental health conditions, GROW and Schizophrenics Anonymous (SA), have a history of using professional leadership for some of their groups. In both instances, researchers, one of whom was involved in both studies, were able to gather data from the groups in order to compare how the professionally led groups differed from the indigenously led groups. The study of professionally led GROW groups occurred twenty years before the study of professionally led SA groups.

The study of GROW groups in Illinois examined the impact of professional leadership or facilitation by gathering social climate and behavioral data on thirty-six professionally led and seventy member-led groups (Toro et al., 1988). The results of the study showed that members in the groups with indigenous leaders perceived their groups to be higher in cohesion, expressiveness, and self-discovery—all three, especially cohesion, being important qualities of effective groups (see chapter 7). In addition, members in those groups reported more agreement comments, information-giving comments, and small talk. It seemed that the presence of professional leaders made members feel less comfortable in the group than when there were no professionals present. In groups with professional leaders, members showed fewer agreement comments, less self-disclosure, less small talk, and less information giving. They also rated the groups as higher in leader control. These findings suggest that professional leaders either intentionally limited effective helper therapy communication or, by their presence, intimidated members, who became less expressive as a result. The researchers were unable to identify any other explanation.

Twenty years later, Salem, Reischl, and Randall (2008) compared outcomes of SA groups, some of which were led by professionals who wanted to form more SA groups in Michigan. The researchers found that professionally led SA groups were successful in increasing the numbers of groups; however, groups led by professionals were more likely to fold within three years. It came out that consumers, when they led chapters, had more choice and control over their groups than when professionals led them. Further, professional leaders did not value members' experiential knowledge, which led some members to feel marginalized and as if there were no roles for them. Members, when asked, were ambivalent about the value of professional leadership. On the one hand, the professionals made it possible for the groups to expand to new areas in the state. Also, they appreciated having paid professionals they could count on. On the other hand, they wished leaders would spend more time "beefing up" (concentrating on) the existing groups and put less time into new group development (p. 188).

The study's authors agreed that leaders needed to spend time beefing up the groups. The short life span of professionally led groups could have had several reasons: lack of investment by members; professional leaders paying too little attention to group process; lack of consumer choice and control preventing members from assuming leadership and investing in the group's survival. Based on this study, the authors recommended member involvement and control as the preferred leadership style as the SA fellowship expanded.

An earlier study (Salem, Gant, & Campbell, 1996) introduced residents of four group homes to SA in order to assess how the linking practices and leadership in the groups affected subsequent participation. Attitudes of group home staff greatly affected whether residents attended meetings. Staff at two of the group homes actively discouraged attendance, and in the other two homes, staff supported attendance; however, once the study period ended, none of the residents continued participation. Factors affecting turnout were severity of illness and residents' ability to identify with the group leader and members. In one case, the leader was an older woman, and the members were all young men. Residents with more serious mental illness also were less able to follow through and benefit from the group. The findings pointed up the importance of staff encouragement for attendance and the importance of group fit (see chapter 9).

All of the studies on professionals as leaders suggest that a professional leader in a self-help group risks deviation from the self-help ethos of valuing experiential knowledge and the helper therapy principle. This would be true unless the professional also shared the problem, as with Dr. Bob in AA. In addition, the leader must value and comprehend the differences among self-help groups, support groups, and therapy groups.

The issue of professional leadership does not arise in twelve-step meetings, because the fellowships have traditions that simply do away with any formal leadership; twelve-step groups do not have *leaders* in the usual sense of the term. Meeting facilitation rotates among members. Helping roles in groups are considered service; certain members take on the group secretary role for a period of time, but this is not group leadership. Twelve-step fellowships all have an inverted hierarchy on the national level, with the individual groups at the top and general service offices at the bottom, which are staffed by rotating members who have no authority. No one person speaks for the fellowship. Tradition Two in AA states: "For our group purpose, there is but one ultimate authority—a loving God as He may express Himself in our group conscience. Our leaders are but trusted servants; they do not govern." Adherence to this tradition guides all twelve-step fellowships (with slight wording changes) to avoid any form of authority within groups or among them. AA's Tradition Eight also speaks to the issue of professional leadership: "Alcoholics Anonymous should remain forever nonprofessional, but our service centers may employ special workers" (AA, 1939/1976, p. 564).

ETHICAL ISSUES RELATED TO LINKING TO SELF-HELP BY PROFESSIONALS

Professional and nonprofessional staff of treatment agencies should use caution when linking consumers to self-help groups in the community. This means that the staff member should be familiar with the group and its program. For example, while one may know twelve-step philosophy in general, one should also be aware of the specific group and its practices. Group members should not interfere with newcomers' medical treatment; should not exploit new members for financial, sexual, or other favors; and should treat newcomers with respect (White & Kurtz, 2006). The staff member responsible for linking someone to a self-help program must, therefore, follow the guidelines in box 5.1 and monitor his or her consumers' contacts with the self-help group.

When linking a new member, professional and nonprofessional staff should be familiar with those whom the self-help group serves in order to be sure that the new person fits the profile for that group. For example, link a drug user to an NA, Cocaine Anonymous, or a similar group and not to an AA group where the drug of choice is alcohol. Link a person with a psychiatric disorder to a group for people with that type of illness and not to an Al-Anon group or an AA group. If a consumer has a dual problem with alcohol and mental illness, link that person to a group for people with dual problems, or be sure to explain to the person the importance of mentioning only the alcohol problem in the alcohol group and only the mental health concern in a group for people with mental health conditions. It is particularly important for a person taking psychiatric drugs to refrain from discussing them in a group for people who want to remain drug-free, such as NA. Likewise, consumers who are being treated with methadone should be linked to a Methadone Anonymous group, not AA or NA, where methadone is often not accepted.

CONCLUSION

This chapter reviewed the demands of forming an independent self-help association and considered those founders who devoted much of their lives to such an endeavor. It suggested that you not reinvent the wheel and turn instead to a national association that already exists for the condition you are addressing. You can find such associations online at the American Self-Help Group Clearinghouse (http://www.mentalhelp.net/selfhelp). The importance of linking people to groups and the ways in which aggressive linking is carried out were discussed, and the ethical issues in linking were summarized.

You may find yourself in the position of wanting a group to form for a particular reason but not wanting or not being able to link the group to a national association of affiliated groups. It might be that the difficulties of the people who need the group are too unusual or too specific for a national group. For example, you could be working with parents of adolescents who have attempted suicide. There are associations for parents whose children have committed suicide but, as far as I know, none for parents whose kids have attempted it and been unsuccessful. The need might be too urgent to wait for a national association to form or respond. You may simply want to begin a support group instead of a group that is part of a national federation. This will be the topic of the next chapter.

REFERENCES

AA. (1939/1976). *Alcoholics Anonymous: The story of how many thousands of men and women have recovered from alcoholism* (3rd. ed.). New York, NY: AA World Services.

Boyer, P. (Unpublished). *The value of Recovery International as an adjunct to psychotherapy.*

Conrad-Garrisi, D. L., & Pernice-Duca, F. (2013). The relationship between sense of mattering, stigma, and recovery: An empirical study of clubhouse participants in the U.S. Midwest. *International Journal of Self-Help and Self-Care, 7*(1), 41–57.

Davidson, L., Tondora, J., Lawless, M. S., O'Connell, M. J., & Rowe, M. (2009). *A practical guide to recovery-oriented practice*. New York, NY: Oxford University Press.

Finn, L., Bishop, B., & Sparrow, N. (2009). Capturing dynamic processes of change in Grow mutual help groups for mental health. *American Journal of Community Psychology, 44*, 302–315.

Humphreys, K. (2004). *Circles of recovery: Self-help organizations for addictions*. Cambridge: Cambridge University Press.

Kaskutas, L. (2009). Alcoholics Anonymous effectiveness: Faith meets science. *Journal of Addictive Diseases, 28*(2), 148–157.

Kelly, J. F., & Moos, R. (2003). Dropout from 12-step self-help groups: Prevalence, predictors, and counteracting treatment influences. *Journal of Substance Abuse Treatment, 24*(3), 241–250.

Keogh, C. (1979). *GROW comes of age*. Sydney: GROW Publications.

Kurtz, L. F. (1984). Linking treatment centers with Alcoholics Anonymous. *Social Work in Health Care, 9*(3), 85–94.

Kurtz, L. F. (1985). Cooperation and rivalry between helping professionals and members of A.A. *Health and Social Work, 10*(2), 104–112.

Kurtz, L. F., Mann, K. B., & Chambon, A. (1987). Linking between social workers and mental health mutual-aid groups. *Social Work in Health Care, 13*(1), 69–78.

Low, A. A. (1943). *Mental illness, stigma and self-help: The founding of Recovery, Inc.* Glencoe, IL: Willett Publishing.

Low, A. A. (1950). *Mental health through will training*. Glencoe, IL: Willett Publishing.

Mandiberg, J. M., & Edwards, M. (2013). Collective identity formation in the mental health clubhouse community. *International Journal of Self-Help & Self-Care, 7*(1), 19–39.

Mechanic, D., & Aiken, L. H. (1989/2011). Improving the care of patients with chronic mental illness. In M. Rowe, M. Lawless, K. Thompson, & L. Davidson (Eds.), *Classics of community psychiatry: Fifty years of public mental health outside the hospital* (pp. 360–367). New York, NY: Oxford University Press.

Moos, R. H., & Moos, B. S. (2006). Participation in treatment and Alcoholics Anonymous: A 16-year follow-up of initially untreated individuals. *Journal of Clinical Psychology, 62*(6), 735–750.

Powell, T., & Perron, B. E. (2010). Self-help groups and mental health/substance use agencies: The benefits of organizational exchange. *Substance Use and Misuse, 45*, 315–329.

Rau, N., & Rau, M. (1971). *My dear ones: The love story of a great physician and his patients*. Englewood Cliffs, NJ: Prentice-Hall.

Salem, D. A., Gant, L., & Campbell, R. (1996). The initiation of self-help groups within residential treatment settings. *Community Mental Health Journal, 24*(4), 419–429.

Salem, D. A., Reischl, T. M., & Randall, K. W. (2008). The effect of professional partnership on the development of a mutual-help organization. *American Journal of Community Psychology, 42*, 179–191.

Salem, D. A., Seidman, E., & Rappaport, J. (1988). Community treatment of the mentally ill: The promise of mutual-help organizations. *Social Work, 33*(5), 403–408.

Smith, A. R. (2007). *The social world of Alcoholics Anonymous: How it works.* Lincoln, NE: iUniverse.

Timko, C., & DeBenedetti, A. (2007). A randomized controlled trial of intensive referral to 12-step self-help groups: One-year outcomes. *Drug and Alcohol Dependence, 90*, 270–279.

Toro, P., Reischl, T., Zimmerman, M., Rappaport, J., Seidman, E., Luke, D. A., et al. (1988). Professionals in mutual help groups: Impact on social climate and members' behavior. *Journal of Consulting and Clinical Psychology, 56*, 631–632.

Torrey, E. F., Kennard, A. D., Eslinger, D., Lamb, R., & Pavle, J. (2010). *More mentally ill persons are in jails and prisons than hospitals: A survey of the states.* Retrieved from http://www.treatmentadvocacycenter.org/storage/documents/final_jails_v_hospitals_study.pdf

White, W., & Kurtz, E. (2006). *Linking addiction treatment and communities of recovery: A primer for addiction counselors and recovery coaches.* Pittsburgh, PA: IRETA.

[S]upport groups involve much more than . . . letting people take turns complaining about things.
KLEIN (2000, p. xi)

6

FACILITATING SUPPORT GROUPS

REMEMBER, SUPPORT GROUPS, as described in chapter 3, differ from self-help groups, and one of the differences is support groups are often led by professionals. The two most frustrating groups I've ever attended were both led by someone who did all the talking. Neither of the leaders understood that the purpose of starting a group is for members to learn from one another—that's why social workers think of such gatherings as mutual-aid groups. To be fair, the nurse in charge of the heart-failure support group for relatives that I attended saw her role as that of educator, which is a legitimate role for a support group facilitator, but lecturing is not the only way to educate. The psychologist at the stress reduction meeting had no excuse for lecturing to his group. I had a lot in common with the other members in both groups, and I was anxious to hear how they handled their relatives with heart problems and the stresses of daily life that caused all of us to have headaches. I attended these groups twenty and thirty years ago, but I still remember how the leaders dominated the groups.

This chapter will focus on how you can be an effective leader or facilitator of a support group. A successful support group may seem so simple to start and maintain that you don't realize the importance of your role. If you are good at it, the participants may not even notice you. But if you make any number of common mistakes, it will be obvious. As in the groups I mentioned above, your members will be frustrated and unhappy—and they may not come back. The life of a group evolves in stages. What follows will discuss those stages in order, beginning with the planning or pre-formation stage.

THE PREFORMATION STAGE

Planning for a group requires that you have answers to several questions before the group begins. Here are six of them.

Who Needs the Group?

One of the most important decisions you have to make is to adopt membership criteria. Your criteria should ensure that only people with something in common qualify for membership. As covered in chapter 3, coming together over commonalities is the essence of a support group. This might simply involve inviting to the group all persons who are members of the local clubhouse or drop-in center. This simplifies criteria by restricting membership to those who meet requirements for belonging to the clubhouse.

You could broaden the criteria by inviting all people in the local community who have a mental health diagnosis. Then you would have to decide what diagnoses to include, who should make the diagnosis, how potential members will prove they qualify, and how you will publicize the group. This gets complicated. The suggestion in the paragraph above limits membership and makes qualifying easy. This second suggestion presents some hurdles to overcome. Think about other ways you could specify the qualifications for membership as you read the rest of this chapter. In general, when someone is actively psychotic, it is better to wait until he or she stabilizes before including that person. This is a decision that will have to be made at the beginning.

What Kind of Program Do You Want?

This could be problem solving, mutual support, or information and education. Do you want to invite guests to speak, or do you want to keep the group closed to just members? Will guests be allowed to come and observe? Will new members be invited to join after the group begins? These decisions determine whether you will have an open group or a closed group.

Do You Have Enough Potential Members?

Support group facilitators with experience suggest that you aim for a minimum of twelve members. To have that many, invite at least twenty people to attend the first meeting. Inevitably, some will not show up. Sometimes your recruitment method will result in having too many attendees for an intimate discussion group. If that should happen, you can include everyone for the first part of the meeting and then split into small discussion groups for the rest of it. Group size is more flexible for support groups than for therapy groups; the latter require about seven members to be therapeutic (Garvin, 1997). Two people can meet for support successfully, just as a large group of twenty can meet and split into smaller pods for supportive interaction.

Will the Group Be Time-Limited, or Will It Continue Indefinitely?

This decision will depend entirely on your core group of members and their goals for the group. Sometimes groups begin with a set number of sessions in mind and then renew at the end of the set period. Other groups come to a natural ending point. This will happen more readily in a group that is closed to new members. A successful open-ended group can go on indefinitely.

Do You Have an Appropriate Meeting Place?

Church basements seem perfect for support and self-help groups. One reason is probably that churches are generous with their space and often have more than they need except for special events and Sundays. Because of the tradition of not accepting outside donations, twelve-step groups pay for their use of space. Churches may have to pay a custodian to open the doors and close them after the meeting. If you cannot pay for your meeting room, you may have to use a room at your agency or clubhouse. This works well for support groups that meet during the agency's open hours. Most important, the space you use should be large enough to be comfortable for members and near transportation for those who have no cars. Even better is the availability of a play room, where children can wait for a parent who cannot afford a babysitter. The meeting room should also offer privacy. You want your group members to feel they can disclose private thoughts and feelings. This will be difficult if the room has no door to close or has no soundproofing. It should be possible to curtain the windows so that no one can look in from outside. The room should be quiet so members can hear one another.

Who Will Lead the Group—a Member or a Professional/Staff Person?

Whomever you choose for this role, there are characteristics that make for a good leader. I found these in a book on support groups by Linda Klein (2000): (1) someone who likes being with people, (2) someone with good verbal skills who can engage people and create group interaction, (3) someone who understands group dynamics, (4) someone who is organized and can create group structure, (5) someone who is a good listener and can accept differences without bias, (6) someone who can question and summarize to build group discussion, (7) someone able to resolve group conflict, (8) someone with a sense of humor, (9) someone committed to the value of peer support. In chapter 5, I discussed professional versus indigenous leadership. For the support group, professional leadership is more common, but what is more important is whether the leader has at least some of the qualities just listed.

LEADERSHIP

A nationwide study of forty-three supportive self-help groups for parents of children with cancer found three leadership patterns that they compared (Yoak & Chesler, 1985). These were groups with only indigenous parent leadership, groups in which the leadership was shared by a professional and a parent, and groups that were led by only a professional. The groups varied. Some were of long standing (5 percent for more than eight years); others were much more recent (67 percent for four and a half years or less). Some groups had varied activities (such as attempts to change the medical system); others had an unvaried single activity, such as group discussion. Most had social activities for members, and members had contacts with one another outside the meetings.

When the three leadership patterns were compared, the professionally led groups were smaller, were less formal, and had shorter lives than those with the other two leadership patterns. The parent-led and shared-leadership groups engaged in more varied activities and were more likely to include parents whose children had died, and these groups lasted longer than the professionally led groups. The short life of the professionally led groups reflects the same finding as in the study of Schizophrenics Anonymous groups reported in chapter 5. It could be that professionals leading support and self-help groups are required by the demands of their agencies to limit group services to people who are still clients of the parent agency. For some reason, their groups die young. To avoid this early death, the study's authors say the professionals should become a resource for the indigenous leadership of the group, foster independence rather than dependence, and solicit member expertise rather than presenting their own. They should be willing to let go when members wish to take over. The shared-leadership pattern in their study suggests a practical option for groups that are first forming, and it is one that easily shifts to full indigenous leadership in the future.

Technically, a support group has a facilitator, not a leader (Miller, 1998). A support group depends on group interaction of a supportive nature. This requires a facilitator who can make that interaction happen in a way that supports members so they will be able to self-disclose what is really going on with them. "A facilitator is more concerned with guiding the process of what happens than the content of what's said and done" (Miller, 1998, p. 30). The facilitator is constantly watching the group's interaction, noting what's said and not said, concentrating on what is happening, and making split-second decisions about when to intervene. It's a difficult skill to learn.

Once you and a potential core group of members have met and have made these important decisions, it is time to arrange for the first meeting and to enter the forming stage of the group.

THE FORMING STAGE

The group's first meeting marks its entry to the forming stage (Tuckman, 1965). The initial stage of group development has been given other labels, such as orientation, but Tuckman's terms for each stage (forming, storming, norming, performing) have captured the attention of group theorists, perhaps because they rhyme and can be remembered that way. Orientation is a good name for this stage, however, because a group formed for people with no prior acquaintance will require some time for members to become familiarized with one another.

Before the first meeting, someone needs to be appointed to greet members at the door to the meeting room. This is pretty standard for support or self-help groups and lets newcomers feel included immediately. Someone must arrange the chairs in the room. The group leader's expectation of what will happen in the group is communicated instantly by the way chairs are arranged. Putting chairs in a circle signals that members will be talking to one another. Chairs set up in rows suggest that members will be sitting silently and listening to someone speak. If a new member walks into the room and pulls a chair away from the circle, this tells you the person is afraid of what might happen in the group, that he or she may be asked to self-disclose, for example, or that he or she might be criticized or expected to reveal more about his or her identity than he or she wants others to know. This fear is normal, although these actions tell you something important.

If your group members already know one another, they will not be experiencing some of the normal concerns of people who enter a group without knowing anyone in it. For a group of strangers, participants will be looking for clues about their fellow members and either consciously or unconsciously deciding if they want to be a part of the group. In the beginning, unless the structure dictates not to do so, the members may direct everything they have to say to the group leader. It's important to redirect them to sharing concerns with one another.

If you want the group to be interactive, the first order of business is introductions, usually first names only. Name tags can be made available for people to wear to help members remember first names, if this is important to the group. In your introductions, you can ask members to say a little about themselves and why they have come to the meeting, but be sure they know that they can pass. When new members enter the group later on, the group should decide how to recognize them. Members may prefer that participants be anonymous, using no names at all. This should be the group's choice.

In the first meeting, the facilitator should let members know what is planned for the group, what the format of the meetings will be, and what they can expect. The facilitator should explain his or her role. Members may be expecting the facilitator to chair the meeting and ask people to speak. Facilitators should explain how they sees their role and what they hope members will do in the group. They should let the group members know that they have the right to pass when it is their turn to speak. Facilitators can say that everyone in the group is there because of something they all have in common—this could be something such as everyone living in a group home or all the members having been in a psychiatric hospital at some time in the past, or all the members being involved in transitional employment. Facilitators should state that they hope members will share their concerns and also their ideas for coping with their situations and that this is the purpose of the group. They should ask members to speak up, say what they think, and offer additional ideas about what the group can discuss and do together. In the first stage or the first meeting, members may be concerned about how safe it will be to share something with the group. A facilitator should make it clear that the group will be a safe place (this means not being forced to talk and not being criticized for what is said) and that no one will be expected to share anything that makes him or her uncomfortable.

By putting the chairs in a circle, you have begun to structure the group. You can go further, by stating your expectations that oral participation will take place in a certain way, such as going around the room without crosstalk (i.e., no one responds directly to the speaker). If you have a large group, the no-crosstalk rule works well, because everyone gets a chance to speak. Responses to what someone says or asks can come from individual members during their own turns to speak.

Another way to structure a group is to have an opening statement read at the beginning of each meeting; this is similar to what self-help groups do. The opening statement can state norms you hope for in the group, such as coming on time, staying to the end of the meeting, using first names only, respecting each member's time to talk, not talking too long, and keeping what is said in the group confidential. It's also important to read or say something about the group's purpose, especially if you have an open group with new members in each meeting.

THE STORMING STAGE

Many groups go through a brief conflict stage (where conflict means disagreement), sometimes called the power-and-control stage, as members struggle to define the group's goals, their relations with one another, and the roles members will play in the group (Forsyth, 2009). Frequently, this struggle over power is directed at the group leader. Low levels of conflict at this stage may simply mean that group members are apathetic about the group; conflict may mean that members take what happens to the group seriously enough to challenge one another or the leader about what the group will discuss, where it will meet, what refreshments will be served, and any number of details. It's important for the facilitator or indigenous leader to understand that this is a normal part of the group's development, accept challenges calmly, and allow the group to consider what it wants to do, what to eat, when and where to meet, and whom to have as members.

I once served on the national board of a civil rights organization that was so internally political that it could barely get beyond deciding on the meeting agenda for a two-day marathon over the weekend. The agenda itself was important, because where an item appeared on the agenda determined whether the group would ever get to it. As I look back on it, I think this group at that time was stuck in the storming stage.

THE NORMING STAGE

In this stage of group development, disagreements fade, and the group becomes cohesive; norms for the group develop spontaneously, perhaps replacing those that the group's facilitator put forth in the beginning. Support groups made up of people with shared life circumstances and struggles naturally move quickly into this stage because they have much in common; if their concerns are at near-crisis levels—facing a diagnosis of serious mental illness, for example—they will value the group and its members highly and cling to what they can learn from one another and to the support they need. The facilitator at this stage can relax and help members offer support to one another.

There will be times when someone opens up, self-discloses, perhaps for the first time, and the group ignores him or her. This is the point at which a sharp facilitator can stop the group, go back to the member who asked for support for the first time, and help the group respond to that person. In this way, the facilitator teaches the group to listen more carefully to others. Because this stage brings more unity and agreement to the group, the professional's role is to monitor and reinforce help-giving support. In Roberts's (1985) assessment of group behavior and member evaluation of group meetings in GROW (a self-help group), she found that a positive evaluation of meetings resulted when there were less negative behaviors and more positive support given by those seen as helpers. Negative behaviors included disagreements, disapproval, and defensiveness. Positive comments were those that gave direct guidance and suggestions and offered encouragement and approval.

THE PERFORMING STAGE

Once the group achieves workable group norms, it reaches the performing stage. This stage is the pinnacle of effectiveness, in which the group regularly accomplishes its goals. Observation of groups has shown that the later stages of a group's life produce more task-focused behaviors than earlier stages (Forsyth, 2009). If it is an open group that admits new members along the way, it will be more difficult for those assembled to reach this stage. For this reason, the inclusion of older members, who have worked through earlier stages of uncertainty and inhibition, will encourage and model performance of group activity.

An ongoing feature in support groups is information exchange. Initially, the group's facilitator brings needed information to the group; in a group for people with mental health conditions, this information might concern medications, other forms of treatment, or availability of community resources. Guest speakers sometimes provide this type of information. As the group enters the performing stage, members themselves become a source of information. Examples of this include experiences in taking a new form of medication, how to get ready for a job interview, and to whom and when to reveal one's mental health diagnosis. Members should also be vocal in asking for information and inviting guest speakers to share new knowledge with the group. The facilitator will encourage and support members' freedom to make choices on their own.

The main goal of the group is member support. The facilitator will have modeled this in earlier stages by responding to member concerns and affirming members when they disclose personal issues. Members should now be making supportive statements and encouraging one another to become active in their recovery and in their efforts to form and pursue new life goals. Members should be able to offer consolation when someone faces difficult times and provide hope through sharing similar experiences and how they coped.

If the group is time-limited, a final stage is termination. At this point, the group members say goodbye and evaluate the experience of the group. Members can pursue other group activities and forge extragroup relationships with the other participants. If the group is open-ended with respect to longevity, it may be time for the facilitator to reduce activity with the group and become more of a consultant, brought in to solve group problems as needed. This can be achieved in stages by reducing oral participation, tapering off the number of meetings attended, and demonstrating a consultant role. The group may want to appoint one of its members to take the facilitator's place, or members may decide to take turns performing that role. At this point, it's a good idea to review the appropriate role of a facilitator and make sure the group understands the difference between a support group and a therapy group.

PROBLEMS THAT COME UP IN SUPPORT GROUPS

Imagine facilitating a group in which one member does all the talking, two others whisper to each other while he or she is babbling on, and another person says nothing. Meanwhile, the member who talks all the time has brought three noisy children to the meeting, and they are running around the room, shrieking and laughing. Does this sound extreme? I hope it does, but I can imagine it. I will now review some of the most common group problems and offer some suggestions on how to deal with them. I will begin with the ones that have been most common in my experience and work down to the least common.

Member Attrition and Absences

The most common problem in support groups is low attendance. There are many possible reasons for it, and correcting or improving attendance requires that you find the source. Here are the most likely reasons:

- *Time and place.* Is the place you are meeting easy to access and safe? Is the time convenient?
- *Too few committed members.* It is typical for support group members to drop in and out of meetings, which means you need to have enough members to make up for frequent absences of others.
- *Lack of similarities among members.* Do members identify with one another enough for group cohesion and commitment to the group?
- *Group safety.* Do members fear something in the group, such as being made to speak, being criticized, or being exposed in some way? If so, these fears need to be put to rest.
- *Negativity.* Members may complain and not get constructive feedback or ideas for coping.

- *A few people who take up all the time.* See below for more discussion of this issue.
- *Lack of child care.* Is there a way to make child care available for members?

The Monopolizer

One, or sometimes two, can monopolize a group. This is a common and difficult problem, partly because people who do this are not aware of it. Even though you may have set the norm for equal exchange among members, this unaware individual has no clue about how long he or she has been talking. One way to deal with it is to introduce a go-around pattern of interaction, with time limits on each person's floor time. Another way is to speak with the dominating person privately and ask him or her to hold back on some comments so others can speak. This is a risky tactic, because people have a low tolerance for criticism; it must be done tactfully. Sometimes you can simply murmur to the individual in the meeting, saying softly, "Wait, let someone else talk."

In a slightly different scenario, two members take on a therapy/therapist exchange while the rest of the group observes passively. The facilitator must intervene in such cases and remind both members that the group is for all members and then ask other members to comment or simply shift to a new topic. In discussing this type of occurrence, Yalom (1970/1995) advises that it is the group leader's responsibility to handle the problem; he or she should not leave it to group members to deal with. In my own experience, group members hold the professional leader accountable for taking care of the group and do not see it as their job to do this for you.

Bringing Outsiders to the Meeting

There should be a firm rule about who is and is not welcome in the meeting. Some groups are very open and welcome anyone. If a group is not this type of group, rules must be made. This is particularly critical when members bring children. Very young children can be disruptive and therefore are not acceptable as guests. Older children can understand what is being said; therefore, they will inhibit participants' willingness to self-disclose; children cannot be expected to keep what they hear and whom they see confidential. A schoolteacher I once knew attended Al-Anon. One day, she entered the group, and there sat one of her students, whose mother had brought him to the meeting with her, having no idea that her fellow group member was a teacher. Children should not be allowed as guests if the group depends on confidentiality. Other adult guests may be acceptable but only if all members agree ahead of time, not when the guest has already arrived. Again, such intrusions can limit self-disclosure and risk confidentiality. Service dogs should be allowed, but other pets can be disruptive, and some members may be allergic to them. If a dog is well behaved and no one objects, it can be a welcome addition.

Inappropriate Emotional Expressions

Unrestrained displays of emotions can disrupt the group and leave the person who loses control, along with others, feeling traumatized and not wanting to return. This is particularly the case if angry feelings are directed at another participant. Remember that safety from criticism is the number one rule for support groups. It is a good idea to make appropriate expression of feeling a goal of the group at the beginning in order to prevent this from happening. It may be acceptable to push for expressing feelings in a therapy group, but this is not the case in a support group. Members may express feelings of grief, loss, happiness, and anger, but they should not be pressed to express feelings with which they are uncomfortable.

Unwillingness to Risk in the Group

The purpose of the support group is helping members cope with stress. This requires that they express their concerns openly so others can respond. Sometimes in such groups, instead of appropriate expression of concerns, the members turn the meeting into a bitching session. Or they talk about the weather, last night's football game, or anything besides the real reason they are there. They are not superficial people, but they are giving superficial attention to the group's purpose. Most people are naturally fearful of self-disclosure, especially in a group of people they do not know well. They may feel that they will be rejected and that the group will ignore them or that they will experience unwanted feelings if they concentrate on serious issues. The group meets so that people with similar difficulties will recognize that they are not alone and that others understand them and that others can help them deal with stress. Group members need to understand that they are there to work on coping with stress; reporting on successes and methods of coping are most appropriate for group discussion. The group's facilitator must help them understand this purpose at the very beginning of the group's first meeting and keep them focused on it through the beginning stages of the group until it reaches the performing stage. Otherwise, the group may not reach that stage.

One way to encourage more serious interaction is to use a structured exercise such as "photovoice exploration" (Cabassa, Nicasio, & Whitley, 2013). With this method, members take pictures that represent a vision of their recovery, and then they bring the photos to the meeting for discussion. This method helps group members "reflect on their recovery, share their experiences with peers, and shape their personal narratives" (p. 841). Other exercises can be used in groups;

however, some exercises may turn the group into a therapy group and distract the it from its support mission.

Leader Burnout

Leader burnout is less likely if the facilitator is a staff person getting paid for the job, but it can happen when one of the members takes on the leader role. Reasons for this could be lack of clarity about group goals, role conflict with a co-leader, or worries about group problems such as too few or too many members. Group leadership by an indigenous member works best if the member-leader genuinely feels that the role supports his or her own recovery and is not simply a burden for which he or she volunteered. It could be how the member-leader gives back what he or she has received through earlier participation. Burnout is less likely if the role is made easier through standard operating procedures such as having an agenda for the meeting, having a consistent pattern of group interaction, lowering group expectations for attendance, and having access to a consultant to go over any problems that come up. Making the leadership role time-limited will also prevent this problem.

Postmeeting Upsets

Participants sometimes come to a meeting boiling over with feelings about something that has happened to them. If the problem takes too much time to process in the meeting, it can be put off until after the meeting, or someone in the meeting can take the individual outside the meeting room to give that person a chance to gather his or her thoughts and cope with the feelings that are boiling over. This is a common method of dealing with individual concerns that go beyond what the group can provide. If the same member comes to the meeting this way week after week, however, it may be that the member needs some additional therapy from a staff person.

Coming to the Meeting Drunk or High on Drugs

Rules about alcohol and drug use should be part of the group's ground rules if you think this may happen. Groups can tolerate some level of drinking and using if it's not obvious; otherwise, members who come to a meeting inebriated or high must be asked to leave in a tactful way. If this becomes a pattern, the individual may be asked not to come back until the use has discontinued, making it clear that it's the behavior being excluded, not the person. A member should be confronted after the meeting and privately to avoid distress for other members who may be frightened to see someone get in trouble. Linking the person to a substance abuse specialist should follow.

Diverse Populations Not Represented

What if you opened your group to a wide range of people, but the only people who showed up were ten European Americans and one African American? What could you do? Research from the 1990s found that when African Americans were the dominant race in groups for substance abusers, they did not drop out, but where the groups had more European Americans dominating the membership, few African Americans stayed involved (Kurtz, 1997). So you know that the one black person may drop out without someone else of similar background joining the group. One way to anticipate this dilemma is to have co-leaders of different racial backgrounds. If that is not possible, another method is to target African American and Latino communities with flyers or asking professional staff in these areas to recommend new members. Your initial publicity about the group should make it seem obviously multiracial by having an illustration depicting people of several races on a sign or flyer.

Confessions of Criminal Behavior

One day, in my group for people who were in a supported-living home, a man stated that he had killed someone. He described how he had stuffed body parts into a trashcan. The group was quiet. No one knew what to say. Finally, we moved on, and I learned later that this man had some delusions and that he frequently made this confession, which no one believed. Whew. That let me off the hook. You may not be so lucky, so you need to be prepared in case someone confesses to something real, such as child abuse. There are some crimes that must be reported, and those cannot fall under the confidentiality guidelines of your agency. The best way to handle this is to let your group know in advance that you cannot keep certain kinds of acts confidential if they are reported in the group. I've added this potential problem last because it does not happen often, but when it does, you must act.

CONCLUSION

This chapter has focused on the role of facilitator in a support group. This role can be filled by a professional, an indigenous group member, or a combination of both. If the group has an indigenous leader, the professional role becomes that of a consultant who comes to the assistance of the group if problems occur. In the next chapter, you will read about what research on self-help and support groups has found are helping factors and more about how the staff person and leader can make the group more useful.

REFERENCES

Cabassa, L. J., Nicasio, A., & Whitley, R. (2013). Picturing recovery: A photovoice exploration of recovery dimensions among people with serious mental illness. *Psychiatric Services, 64*(9), 837–842.

Forsyth, D. R. (2009). *Group dynamics* (5th ed.). Belmont, CA: Wadsworth/Cengage.

Garvin, C. D. (1997). *Contemporary group work* (3rd ed.). Boston, MA: Allyn & Bacon.

Klein, L. L. (2000). *The support group sourcebook: What they are, how you can find one, how they can help you*. New York, NY: Wiley.

Kurtz, L. F. (1997). *Self-help and support groups: A handbook for practitioners*. Thousand Oaks, CA: Sage.

Miller, J. E. (1998). *Effective support groups: How to plan, design, facilitate and enjoy them*. Fort Wayne, IN: Willowgreen Publishing.

Roberts, L. J. (1985, August). Measures of self-help group quality: Observer and participant views. Paper presented at the 93rd Annual Convention of the American Psychological Association, Los Angeles, CA.

Tuckman, B. (1965). Developmental sequence in small groups. *Psychological Bulletin, 63*(6), 384–399.

Yalom, I. D. (1970/1995). *The theory and practice of group psychotherapy* (4th ed.). New York, NY: Basic Books.

Yoak, M., & Chesler, M. (1985). Alternative professional roles in health care delivery: Leadership patterns in self-help groups. *Journal of Applied Behavioral Science, 21*(4), 427–444.

It's not the sharing of woes that compels attachment to the group; it's the sharing of recovery.
KURTZ (see below)

7

HOW RECOVERY GROUPS HELP

PEOPLE ATTEND RECOVERY groups at least as often as they seek professional therapy, which raises the question of why. What is it that these groups do that helps with the conditions from which members suffer? As long ago as 1970, Irvin Yalom identified helping factors in therapy groups, most of which he says can also be found in other kinds of groups. In the preface to his text, Yalom says that self-help groups are cousins to therapy groups and that certain helping factors are the core mechanisms of change. These are limited in number, but "intrinsic to the therapeutic process" and found in many small groups, not just psychotherapy groups (Yalom, 1970/1995, p. xii). Investigations of group helping factors over the years have found that there are about twelve. Studies of self-help and support groups point toward three factors especially that should exist in virtually any recovery group: group cohesiveness, universality, and instillation of hope.

COHESIVENESS

Group cohesion is higher in self-help groups than in psychotherapy groups, according to social climate studies by Moos, Finney, and Maude-Griffon (1993) (see chapter 8 for more on social climate). According to one study, AA groups that rate high in cohesion produce more successful outcomes than groups with less cohesion (Rynes, Tonigan, & Rice, 2013). Cohesiveness, defined as having a sense of "groupness" and esprit de corps, is the foundation for the following group effects on members: willingness to self-disclose; conveyance of warmth, acceptance, and friendship to one another; and openness to new ways of looking at things. Yalom viewed cohesiveness among group members as the analog to relationship with an individual therapist; research shows that it is the relationship with the therapist that is the key to successful therapy; therefore, group cohesiveness may be a key to success for members' achievement of group goals. Esprit de corps stems from the extent to which members like one another, are attracted to the group, and wish to remain part of it. The high cohesiveness of recovery self-help groups comes from the strength of group norms, the similarity of member goals for the group, and the openness of interpersonal expressions of liking for one another. For anyone, but especially for people suffering from a stigmatizing condition, being accepted as part of a group has tremendous value and strengthens attachments to the group.

UNIVERSALITY

The essence of a self-help or support group lies in its gathering of people with a particular identity, a common problem, one core concern—such as alcoholism, depression, overeating, or schizophrenia. When people experience a terrible secret or a stigmatizing condition, they wrongly but wrenchingly feel completely alone, unique in their unworthiness. The late Dan Anderson called a variation of this the "very special worm" feeling. "The alcoholic," he would say, "doesn't just feel special, and he doesn't just feel that he's a worm; the alcoholic feels that he is a very special worm" (Anderson, personal communication). While the feeling of specialness may uniquely belong to the alcoholic, anyone who has experienced a mental health condition can identify with the uncomfortable sense of strangeness and isolation that comes with not fitting in.

An Al-Anon member talked about the feeling of similarity that came with her attendance at an Al-Anon group. "It's a closeness. I could talk to my best friend, and she wouldn't know what I was talking about," she said about the universal experiences of members in her group (Kurtz, 1994, p. 300). Families of people who abuse substances isolate themselves in hopes of covering up the terrible secret of addiction in their family. This adds to the feeling of uniqueness. It is true that most of their acquaintances, friends, and extended family members do not understand what they are experiencing. They find this understanding in the family groups. This is one of the reasons for a twelve-step program's singleness of purpose; that is, groups are open only to those who qualify as having the problem shared by other members of the group.

INSTILLATION OF HOPE

It's not the sharing of woes that compels attachment to the group; it's the sharing of recovery. Older members, telling their stories of what they used to be like and what they are like now, give hope. "Here's how bad I was, and now here's how I've changed since being in this group." Veteran members share their experience, strength, and hope.

Newcomers often enter a recovery group unwillingly, without hope, without the motivation to lick their habit or to share their imperfections with others. Hope for something better is essential to getting them to come back and form an attachment to the group. Seeing happy faces, hearing pleasant conversation, feeling comradeship inspires hopefulness. Hope comes from observing success; giving people the ability to experience hope has been defined as one of the hallmarks of the recovery concept (Walsh, 2013).

The discussion that follows will look at helping factors found through research on recovery groups. This will lead to suggestions for how these helping elements can be fostered by group leaders. First, we discuss the factors that are present in both self-help and support groups: giving support, imparting information, giving a sense of belonging, giving a sense of mattering, and learning to cope.

SUPPORT

What is support? I define it as a combination of words and silent attention, personal disclosure, and empathy. It can encompass almost all of the other helping factors to be discussed; it is the primary purpose of a support group. For a group to be supportive, it must first allow members to express themselves openly enough for others to comprehend their situations. Next, it must make time and encourage others to share experiences so the first person to speak can see that he or she is not alone. Ben Gottlieb wrote in 1982 that support encompasses learning to cope, having a sense of community, helping to cope with public attitudes, getting factual information, attaining a spirit of hope, acquiring self-confidence, and meeting others with similar problems.

A study by Roberts and others (1999) of communication in meetings of GROW, a mental health self-help group, found that supportive, help-giving comments, direct guidance, and suggestions correlated with positive meeting evaluations by members. In contrast, negative comments and probing personal questions resulted in negative meeting evaluations. Support was crucial to success. People feared being criticized or pushed to reveal too much.

The finding that probing questions led to negative evaluations of the group bears examination. People open up when they see that the group is safe (in that it will not cause emotional pain or feeling foolish), and they see this by watching other members open up willingly and without judgmental reactions. Pressure to expose participants should be avoided. Even if the one being pressured is an old-timer who can take it, the newcomer does not know that. What newcomers see going on with others in the group will be what they expect will happen to them, and if they imagine it to be frightening or painful, they will not open up and may not come back. The group must first and foremost be a safe place for expressing feelings without judgment.

GIVING INFORMATION AND ADVICE

The second most obvious helping factor in self-help and support groups is imparting information and advice. In some groups, outside guests bring in expert knowledge. In my online support group, we rely on professional expertise on canine neurology and endocrine functions to understand what is going on with our epileptic dogs. This advice is connected with links on the website and making individual consultations with experts possible when necessary. But most of the time, we rely on the day-to-day experiences of fellow members who have been living with the illness longer than we have and who go online daily to respond in case of a crisis.

Groups such as those of the National Alliance on Mental Illness sponsor a number of activities: (1) open meetings in which speakers give professional information about treatment strategies and medications, (2) conferences that offer forums for discussion, (3) newsletters that publish important new knowledge, (4) lobbying and other political actions in support of policy for mental health services, and (5) support groups in which participants share their experiential knowledge.

Experiential knowledge is a term that was coined by Thomasina Borkman in 1976 to describe a "critical component that distinguishes self-help groups from their professionally-based equivalents" (p. 446). She defines it as "truth learned from personal experience with a phenomenon rather than truth acquired by discursive reasoning" (p. 446). It is the wisdom gained from personal experience in the world, know-how that is concrete, specific, and commonsensical, based on actual experience, "unique, limited, and more or less representative of the experience of others who have the same problem" (p. 446). Along with this, there is the competence and skill of being able to cope with that shared common experience. Not all with the same experience history will have learned to cope. They may know full well what the experience is like but still be at a loss regarding how to handle it. That coping knowledge is passed from one successful member to others in the group.

The group may invite professional experts to its meetings to impart their professional knowledge and expertise, deriving from their scientific study of the condition and their background of applying specialized knowledge to the treatment and rehabilitation of the individual with the condition. This might be particularly true with knowledge of current medications for schizophrenia or information on the treatment being offered at the local mental health center. In contrast, the person with experiential knowledge may know, from a different angle, what it's like to apply for emergency admission to the hospital on a Saturday at midnight. Professional expertise is theoretical, scientific, and bureaucratic, whereas experiential knowledge is pragmatic, here-and-now, action-oriented, and holistic.

Experiential knowledge is imparted in informal go-around contributions of the members present. In AA and other twelve-step groups, members share experiential knowledge in the "lead"; that is, an individual stands before the group and tells his or her story of recovery from addiction. In Recovery International, members offer panel discussions on situations in which they spotted themselves working up angry or fearful tempers and how they handled them using recovery principles. Other activities of the self-help community reinforce learning experiences for persons with problem conditions, helping to convert them from a victim/sufferer identity to a recovering survivor identity.

With both types of knowledge, ineffective, inaccurate formulations of the "truth" are constantly tested by experience. New treatments will replace those of professionals whose methods fail the rigors of both theory and research (psychiatric theories of parent-induced schizophrenia, for example), and self-help groups with extreme or outmoded programs will die from lack of new members.

ACHIEVING A SENSE OF BELONGING

People with active addictions have given up or seriously compromised their membership in most of the groups to which they formerly belonged—family, work, and social groups. Once into the life of addiction, they become members of drinking circles or solitary drinkers with no group affiliation at all. People with a psychiatric disability likewise have trouble fitting into everyday social life where their symptoms and other limitations are not understood or accepted. Participation in recovery groups gives these individuals a place to belong. Julian Rappaport's research on GROW, a mental health group, revealed that a group like this, a self-help group, is not an alternative treatment; it is, rather, a normative structure like a family or a voluntary association (Rappaport, 1993). Members are not clients; they are people living lives. And attending a meeting of such a group is not a dose of treatment; it's part of a way of life. Achieving a sense of belonging to a self-help community begins the process of identity change. As a member of a self-help community, one need not graduate but simply moves from being a newcomer to being a veteran member who brings a message of hope to others, in that way creating and maintaining the community.

MAKING A DIFFERENCE AND HAVING A SENSE OF MATTERING

Membership in a self-help or support group provides the participant with a way of making a difference. Kurtz (1982) describes AA's beginning. Bill Wilson and Dr. Bob Smith, the founders, began by approaching a hospitalized alcoholic and asking him to listen to their stories. They told this first recruit, known as "the man on the bed," that they were talking to him for their own sake, so they could stay sober. His response was to listen, because, he said, he didn't mind listening if it would help them. Everyone else wanted to help him, but his pride had prevented him from listening to them. He became the third member of the fledgling AA group.

Kurtz quotes R. D. Laing, who said of the therapeutic approach, "A prototype of the other as giver but not receiver, unresponsive or impervious, tends to generate in self a sense of failure.... Frustration becomes despair when the person begins to question his own capacity to mean anything to anyone" (Kurtz, 1982, p. 59).

In every group, members make a difference for one another, because without them, the group could not go on. For people with negative self-identities, this could be the only place where they see their presence being needed or missed. Making a difference is another way of having a sense of mattering (Conrad-Garrisi & Pernice-Duca, 2013). A sense of mattering is defined as the feeling that others depend on us and are interested in us and concerned with our fate. Having a sense of mattering to others is crucial to reducing negative identities and recovering from psychiatric disability.

TEACHING COPING METHODS

People with mental illnesses and/or addictions often encounter situations in which they cannot cope, either with the intensity of their own feelings or with interpersonal struggles. This is also true for their families. Take the case of the spouse of an active addict. He or she is entangled with the addicted person in the sense that their lives are bound together in parenting, housekeeping, wage earning, and many additional small but important matters. The addict's problem presents a hindrance in getting things done, and the spouse encounters realistic threats to his or her way of life. One must find a way to cope with this reality.

Al-Anon Family Groups teaches the art of detachment. The nondrinking spouse must take over the functions that the drinking spouse has either abandoned or bungled. The impulse is to rant and rave at the underfunctioning person, but this solves nothing. Detachment means letting go of it. It involves forming a shell in which one does what one can and then withdraws those efforts when they are of no use. It is difficult to make this adjustment, but it is essential to the peace of mind of the family. Many Al-Anon meetings focus at least part of the time on describing this process in action and reflecting on its importance. When members relate their stories, they describe how they detach.

Another example is how families of people with schizophrenia and/or addiction must learn to communicate with reduced intensity of feeling. Symptoms increase when feelings run high; drug users are used to anesthetizing feelings, so they want to drink or use when feelings rise. Intense feelings stir people up, and for people who are not able to cope well with feelings, their expression accentuates problems. A family member I spoke with once told me: "My sponsor told me that when I talked to him, just keep to the facts. Before that, I would have been crying and screaming and yelling and everything. So I was talking to him really factual, and part of me was looking at this and saying, is this really me?" (Kurtz, 1994, p. 304).

Members of Recovery International cope with what they prefer to call their nervous problems by learning to use a number of cognitive strategies, by using a different vocabulary to characterize situations that typically get them into a working-up frame of mind. Each person develops insight into the kind of thinking that affects him or her uniquely. These are situations that become a strong link to the working-up process for that one individual; recognizing strong links helps them to spot temperamental situations more quickly. A typical example is when someone reacts in anger to an e-mail message and, without thinking, responds to it right away with an angry retort—so easy to do by e-mail. One learns that angry reactions to e-mail should send up a red flag to wait and think it over before responding.

The helping factors just discussed could apply to any recovery group, whether it is a small support-type group or a more complex self-help association. Those discussed next are typically found in the larger, more multidimensional self-help programs whose members hope for behavioral or system change, rather than the simpler support-type groups. These change-oriented features include identity transformation, empowerment, insight, reframing, and the formation of a new way of life.

IDENTITY TRANSFORMATION

The newcomer enters a group sponsored by the association, recognizes what he or she has in common with those already there, and identifies with the others. Identifying is important and begins the new member's fit into the group. Group fit is an essential aspect in an early stage of participation. Some large associations such as Alcoholics Anonymous mount so many groups in larger population centers that they can have special groups for members that enhance the likelihood that a newcomer will fit in (e.g., young people, lesbians, women, doctors, or atheists). This also explains why it is so important that mixtures of problem identities are excluded or at least suppressed. A member who has alcoholism and also schizophrenia is asked to speak about only the alcohol side of the problem in a generic AA group. Dual-problem groups offer a way to tackle two issues at once.

Once involved in the group, the newcomer acquires characteristics of older members' ways of being. The newcomer's evolving story reveals his or her identity transformation in the recovery group. He or she is no longer sick but is recovering (Borkman, 1999). In the same way, the clubhouse community movement provides members with opportunities for collective identity formation and redefinition (Mandiberg & Edwards, 2013). Just being called a member begins that process.

In the past, accepting a label was seen as negative, but for many, the label allows them to understand what is wrong and points in the direction of finding what is right. In writing about a family's burden of having a relative with a mental health condition, David A. Karp (2001) found that the diagnosis for some was like an epiphany; finally, they had a plausible explanation for their difficulties, an illness reality. If it could be named, something could be done about it. In groups for people with bipolar disorder, members attempted to repair their identities by identifying well-known, successful people with the bipolar diagnosis—another example of redefinition.

Members of Schizophrenics Anonymous talk about how much it means to them to see other people with that diagnosis tell a room full of people about their illness and how they are recovering: "They know what it's like to hear voices that nobody else hears, or they know what it's like to get paranoid and think the whole world's talking about you and be convinced of it and not be able to shake the feeling; even though people reassure you, it doesn't mean a thing" (Randall & Salem, 2007, pp. 192–193).

As Randall and Salem note, schizophrenia is so negative that because of the stigma, newly diagnosed people rarely meet other people who claim the diagnosis; therefore, they cannot see role models who have overcome it and are successfully recovering. The organization counters this when it provides member stories, literature, and videos by and of successfully recovering people with a schizophrenia diagnosis.

BECOMING EMPOWERED

The first sign of empowerment is when one takes action on behalf of oneself. It comes with belief in oneself and growth of self-confidence, usually within a group of other people with something in common. Some dislike the twelve-step philosophy of powerlessness within the individual and recognition of a "power greater than ourselves." But that powerlessness is only over what cannot be controlled, the one drink that leads to more, the self-importance based on nothing real. Bateson (1971/2000, pp. 309–337) wrote that accepting powerlessness over those things that cannot be changed is the first step toward empowerment. Trying to have power over something uncontrollable is futile. By joining with others, the member is empowered to work toward both social change and individual change.

A member of Schizophrenics Anonymous remarked: "It [SA] makes me feel like I've got something to give back to a system that's given me a purpose" (Randall and Salem, 2007, p. 195). Asked about community involvement and political activity, an AA member said: "There are times when I'm doing some form of community work and I realize that all the time I've spent at AA meetings sitting, listening, and learning was done to benefit the experience I'm having at that moment. My ability to handle that experience is a result of many, many hours of just sitting at AA meetings and just listening" (Kurtz & Fisher, 2003, p. 889).

ACHIEVING INSIGHT

Researchers have found that insight comes more easily to members in groups when they have accepted the problem—mental disability, addiction, compulsive disorder—than for those who deny it. They begin to recognize their inner dynamics by seeing themselves reflected in other group members (Goodman & Jacobs, 1994). Insights come about slowly over time and are not pressured by a brief professional therapy regime that demands insight and progress before the insurance runs out. Smith (2007, p. 106) quotes a woman in her sixties who almost drank at Christmastime after she had been in AA for three years: "A woman invited me to a party, and the alcohol was flowing. I figured I might try to have just one glass of punch. But something came over me just as I was about to pour it. I thought, *I'm an alcoholic... an alcoholic... and this could kill me!* I left the party and drove to an Alkathon. And all the way over I kept saying, *thank you God.*"

How easy it was for her to rationalize drinking that one little cup of punch, and how narrow was her escape from this sudden impulse. It took three years of meetings for this woman to have insight into how "cunning, baffling, and powerful" alcoholism can be (AA, 1939/1976, pp. 58–59).

REFRAMING

Reframing or cognitive restructuring consists of making a shift in the way one sees something. Achieving a new way of looking at what is wrong leads to new ideas about how to correct it. The classic example in the self-help world is Abraham Low's method of will training (Low, 1950). Members reframe symptoms and learn new vocabulary. Low believed that former patients of the psychiatric hospital used a symptomatic idiom to work themselves into a nervous collapse. Further, when his former patients worked themselves up into angry or fearful temper, they used the temperamental lingo. Will training teaches group members to use recovery language. They don't think of themselves as having psychiatric diagnoses; they describe themselves as subject to temper, either angry or fearful. They learn to conquer episodes of temper by reframing events that typically lead to symptoms. For example, a woman gets worked up over domestic disputes and typically voices angry feelings followed by a long period of not speaking to her spouse. Reframing allows the woman to see the same situation as something merely irritating that normally happens in married life. The situation is uncomfortable but not serious. This allows the injured spouse to conquer emotion and show group-mindedness, thus preserving peace in the home. The Recovery method is all about learning and using this language to reframe situations that may be trivial at first but can become dangerous to the recovery process if allowed to build up.

Another example of reframing comes from family groups in which relatives of people with serious mental illness or alcoholism first enter feeling they are somehow to blame for the relative's condition and that they should learn to control it. One of the first things they learn in the family group is the three Cs: you didn't cause it, you can't cure it, and you can't control it. In his book on family burden, Karp (2001) adds a fourth C: all you can do is cope with it. This set of factual statements easily reframes family members' feelings of guilt and need to control; the last one points them in the direction of what to do.

This fits with another powerful reframing example: seeing addiction or mental illness as neither a sin nor someone's fault. It is a disease. For twelve-step people, the disease is multifaceted: physical, mental, and spiritual (as mentioned in the "Big Book," AA, 1939/1976, p. 64). Although AA did not originate the disease concept of alcoholism, it did perceive alcoholism as a type of malady. This perspective replaced the painful feeling of being weak-willed, which was how most alcoholics felt and how most people thought of them. Thinking that stopping addictive behavior is only a matter of willpower leads people to think that they should be able to continue the behavior and simply try harder to stop before it gets out of control. Once the behavior starts, however, the disease takes over.

A woman in AA said this: "I couldn't allow myself to think I was anything so terrible as an alcoholic. Then after going to some meetings, I learned that alcoholism was a disease. What that meant was that I could be an alcoholic and learn to resolve problems in healthy ways... and I can do that as long as I don't take a drink" (Smith, 2007, pp. 91–92).

NEW WAY OF LIFE AND REDEFINITION OF SELF

Rappaport (1993) found, after listening to the personal stories of GROW members, that their life stories reflected the group's community narrative. Mutual-help group member narratives do not resemble typical psychiatric patient narratives but are more like the narratives associated with church members. Identity formation takes place in the context of a voluntary community; personal change can be understood as a change in lifestyle rather than as a "treatment outcome" (Rappaport, 1993). Humphreys (2000) found the same was true for stories in AA. As newcomers begin to tell how they came to the program, they tailor a personal narrative to conform to the community narrative. If they happen to deviate from the accepted understanding, they find themselves being ignored until they learn how to fit their story into one that is consonant with the community.

In some self-help fellowships, such as many of the twelve-step programs, the number of groups available in a particular locale makes it possible to attend a meeting every day and at every time of day. These formal meetings are supplemented with the availability of Alano Clubs. These are private clubs open to all local twelve-steppers, where meetings and informal socializing take place daily from early morning to evening. A recovering man interviewed by Annette Smith (2007, p. 34) reflected the feeling of many members: "This is my family now. My folks washed their hands of me a long time ago. I've been through four marriages. I do want to get back with my kids someday. But for now, I get what I need from the people here. They're the ones that taught me how to live."

Smith's research shows how AA conforms to the concept of social world organization with a highly permeable structure, where members have a common bond, but membership is fluid and voluntary. "There are no official membership rolls, dues or organizational hierarchies" (2007, p. 7). The social world exhibits shared values, a common language, and formal and informal social interactions in which it expands to include other social organizations and crosses boundaries with other social worlds. Members can maintain different levels of involvement in the world, as will be discussed further in chapter 8.

Attending a few self-help group meetings does not lead to a new way of life, unless it leads to immersion in the culture of the fellowship. For example, clubhouse culture, such as that of Fountain House and others that follow its example, gives members a chance for new lifestyles. Individualized services, such as traditional psychotherapy, case management, and dyadic relationships with staff, do not provide opportunities for identity formation as part of a community; thus, they sacrifice the advantage of collective relationships that buffer stigma and discrimination (Mandiberg & Edwards, 2013). The freedom of community life is highly valued by people with mental health conditions, even when it often offers little in the way of socialization and relationship building (Davidson, Hoge, Merrill, Rakfeldt, & Griffith, 1995/2011). Adding a self-help or clubhouse opportunity for people with disabilities in the community gives them opportunities for relationship building.

ENCOURAGING HELPING FACTORS

Table 7.1 lists the helping factors just covered and briefly highlights ways to encourage these factors. Although the list is long, common themes point to leadership strategies for strengthening group processes favorable to recovery. Intrinsic to all of them is the importance of making the group attractive to members, both to support newcomers so that they come back and continue recovery and to hold on to members over lengthy periods. The latter serves several purposes. Veteran members teach coping skills and show by their lengthy recovery times that there is hope for those just entering recovery. Recovery takes time; it does not happen overnight and may continue for a lifetime. The more the group connects with a larger network, the more it can offer opportunities for individuals to make a difference and form new identities. Encouraging member contributions of experiential knowledge is as important as expert information; however, feeling safe in the group is necessary for members to be willing to risk self-exposure.

AVOIDING UNHELPFUL FACTORS

Self-help and support groups can be tricky, and it's unwise to assume that nothing bad will happen in them. As a group leader, practitioner, or recovery coach, you need

TABLE 7.1
ENCOURAGING HELPING FACTORS

Helping Factor	Ways of Encouraging
Cohesiveness	Encourage positive reception to newcomers; set strong norms of friendliness.
Universality	Keep membership similar in problem type and goals.
Instillation of hope	Encourage stories of success; make time for everyone to speak.
Giving support	Encourage free expression and positive comments; discourage probing questions and criticism of any kind.
Imparting information	Use go-around communication to encourage sharing experiential knowledge.
Achieving a sense of belonging	Welcome newcomers; hang on to old-timers who offer hope and sponsorship.
Making a difference	Let members know they matter to the group; reinforce members helping newcomers; let newcomers know they help by being helped.
Teaching coping methods	Encourage successful members to share their wisdom.
Identity transformation	Pay attention to group fit; help members see themselves as recovering rather than sick and their illness as only one facet of themselves.
Empowerment	Encourage stories of times when members took action in their own or others' behalf.

to be aware of some mistakes that can happen in groups and how to avoid them. Otherwise, you may discourage participation or even do harm. You will need to cultivate norms that ensure safety from criticism in your group and prevent harmful interactions. These warnings fall into six categories: harmful and misguided advice, overwhelming the group with excessive intensity of feeling, unkind confrontations or personal attacks, exposing members to frightening conditions, trying to do therapy in a group not intended for that purpose, and inappropriate efforts to begin relationships with other members. Most of these problems can be handled by setting ground rules and expressing them clearly, orally and in writing.

To prevent harmful advice, my online canine epilepsy group leaders made it clear when I joined that I should only respond to others by stating my own experience. For example, I cannot say, "You should give your dog this drug" or "You should increase the dose of the medication." Instead, I can say, "When my dog had that happen, this is what I did." The group's leaders had special training and were prepared to give more complex information by referring members to the group's archives. I have been a member for many years. It happened once that a member was giving advice to other members outside the group, in private e-mails. When the leaders found out, they removed that member from the e-mail list. This simple ground rule prevents members from giving misguided advice or appearing to practice medicine without a license, and it is easy to explain and remember. Ground rules like this one should be provided when members enter the group, and reminders should become part of the introduction at every meeting if it's a face-to-face group.

Excessive feelings displayed in a group meeting can frighten other members and end up making the person who is allowed to express them feel embarrassed later. Again, a ground rule can be made that limits such expressions in a meeting. People who have difficulty with feelings, theirs or others', become uncomfortable and frightened when someone loses control. A leader or experienced member can take charge when something like this happens and can usher the person outside, where he or she can calm down before returning.

Confrontations and personal attacks rank as the number one no-no in small groups. I have only experienced something like this once in all my years of observing and sitting in on meetings of all kinds. This was in an e-mail support group that was anything but supportive. The leaders of the group were so antagonistic to new members that people were afraid to post a question on the list. I received my share of abuse before giving up and exiting this particular group, also a group for people with sick dogs, this time concerning orthopedic surgery.

One way to keep the group supportive is for the leader to model supportive responses. In addition, a typical communication pattern is for members to go around the room, with each person taking a set time to speak. Feedback about something a speaker has offered comes when the person commenting takes his or her turn, and then the comment is addressed to the group rather that to the individual. The exchange would go something like the following fictional account:

> Speaker A: I've been so afraid that my dog is going to die that I've had trouble sleeping at night. Last night, I took three sleeping pills before I could sleep.

Several turns go by.

> Speaker B: I've had the problem of worrying about my dog and thinking he may die when his breathing is funny or that he will have a seizure. I've taken sleeping pills before, but now I try not to, because my doctor warned me against doing that.

In this exchange, the speaker B gently confronts speaker A by sharing what her doctor said when she used sleeping pills, rather than directly telling speaker A that she shouldn't take sleeping pills. Also, she starts out by saying that she has done the same thing.

Not exposing members to frightening conditions involves having some control over who enters the group. An example would be having a newcomer attend a group when the newcomer has not been stabilized during a psychotic episode. I once made the mistake of accepting a new member whose illness was not stable for a support group in my mental health agency. In one-on-one talks with him, he was engaging, not psychotic, and seemed like a perfect fit for the group. But I did not know him well enough. In his first meeting, he became manic and began rambling in a loud voice about his religious ideas. After the group meeting had ended, the regular members asked me not to let him return. They were not so much frightened as they were protective of the stability of the group. They saw his presence as a threat to that stability and the future of the group, and they were right.

Efforts to do therapy in a group not intended for that purpose might happen if a new group leader takes over a support group without being clear on its purpose or if a member misunderstands the mission of the group. The new leader might engage a group member in a one-on-one exchange about the member's problem or give interpretations of member dynamics and not realize that the group is for member exchanges of experiential knowledge where they help one another cope. In general, group leaders do not dominate support or self-help groups. Their role is to encourage participation by all members.

Inappropriate efforts to establish relationships with other members present group leaders with a difficult situation. Support groups, self-help groups, and clubhouses offer places for people to establish social ties. Social encounters are inappropriate when they expose people to others who try to harass or scam them. Ground rules need to be in place to let all members know that these kinds of overtures are unacceptable and that anyone who violates that rule will be asked not to come back. Large self-help fellowships such as AA or NA experience their share of this kind of thing—participants who attempt to seduce new members, sell drugs after the meeting, or ask to borrow money. Veteran members and sponsors try to prevent this from happening, and program literature warns against it, but the programs are so large that it is hard to prevent.

CONCLUSION

The list of helping factors is long and may seem daunting to a new group participant. Keep in mind that most of them happen spontaneously as the group meets and members share their everyday experiences. As a leader, your role is to make the group a benign place and to ensure that certain hindrances to free expression and self-disclosure do not happen. In the next chapter, there are some specific recommendations that can help you do that.

This list of warnings concludes the chapter on helping and unhelpful factors in group life. The next chapter addresses three other group characteristics: social climate, group philosophy and teachings, and group structure. These three elements shape how a group helps individual members and also how it maintains itself as an attractive place for people to meet.

REFERENCES

AA. (1939/1976). *Alcoholics Anonymous: The story of how many thousands of men and women have recovered from alcoholism* (3rd ed.). New York, NY: AA World Services.

Bateson, G. (1971/2000). *Steps to an ecology of the mind: Collected essays in anthropology, psychiatry, evolution, and epistemology.* Chicago, IL: University of Chicago Press.

Borkman, T. (1976). Experiential knowledge: A new concept for the analysis of self-help groups. *Social Service Review, 50*, 445–456.

Borkman, T. (1999). *Understanding self-help mutual aid: Experiential learning in the commons.* New Brunswick, NJ: Rutgers University Press.

Conrad-Garrisi, D. L., & Pernice-Duca, F. (2013). The relationship between sense of mattering, stigma, and recovery: An empirical study of clubhouse participants in the U.S. Midwest. *International Journal of Self-Help and Self-Care, 7*(1), 41–57.

Davidson, L., Hoge, M. A., Merrill, M. E., Rakfeldt, J., & Griffith, E. E. H. (1995/2011). The experience of long-stay inpatients returning to the community. In M. Rowe, M. Lawless, K. Thompson, & L. Davidson (Eds.), *Classics of community psychiatry: Fifty years of public mental health outside the hospital* (pp. 440–451). New York, NY: Oxford University Press.

Goodman, G., & Jacobs, M. K. (1994). The self-help mutual-support group. In A. Fuhriman & G. Burlingame (Eds.), *Handbook of group psychotherapy: An empirical and clinical synthesis* (pp. 489–526). New York, NY: John Wiley.

Gottlieb, B. H. (1982). Mutual-help groups: Members views of their benefits and of roles for professionals. *Prevention in Human Services, 1*(3), 55–68.

Humphreys, K. (2000). Community narratives and personal stories in Alcoholics Anonymous. *Journal of Community Psychology, 28*(5), 495–506.

Karp, D. A. (2001). *The burden of sympathy: How families cope with mental illness.* New York, NY: Oxford University Press.

Kurtz, E. (1982). Why A.A. works: The intellectual significance of Alcoholics Anonymous. *Journal of Studies on Alcohol, 43*(1), 38–80.

Kurtz, L. F. (1994). Self-help groups for families with mental illness or alcoholism. In T. J. Powell (Ed.), *Understanding self-help organizations: Frameworks and findings* (pp. 293–313). Thousand Oaks, CA: Sage.

Kurtz, L. F., & Fisher, M. (2003). Participation in community life by AA and NA members. *Contemporary Drug Problems, 30*, 875–904.

Low, A. (1950). *Mental health through will training.* Glencoe, IL: Willett Publishing.

Mandiberg, J. M., & Edwards, M. (2013). Collective identity formation in the mental health clubhouse community. *International Journal of Self-Help & Self-Care, 7*(1), 19–39.

Moos, R. H., Finney, J., & Maude-Griffon, P. (1993). The social climate of self-help mutual support groups: Assessing group implementation, process, and outcome. In B. S. McCrady and W. R. Miller (Eds.), *Research on Alcoholics Anonymous: Opportunities and alternatives* (pp. 251–270). New Brunswick, NJ: Rutgers Center for Alcohol Studies.

Randall, K. W., & Salem, D. A. (2007). Mutual-help groups and recovery: The influence of settings on participants' experience of recovery. In R. O. Ralph & P. W. Corrigan (Eds.), *Recovery in mental illness: Broadening our understanding of wellness* (pp. 173–205). Washington, DC: American Psychological Association.

Rappaport, J. (1993). Narrative stories, personal stories, and identity transformation in the mutual-help context. *Journal of Applied Behavioral Science, 29*, 239–256.

Roberts, L. J., Salem, D., Rappaport, J., Luke, D. A., Toro, P. A., & Seidman, E. (1999). Giving and receiving help: Interpersonal transactions in mutual-help meetings and psychosocial adjustment of members. *American Journal of Community Psychology, 27*, 841–869.

Rynes, K. N., Tonigan, J. S., & Rice, S. L. (2013). Interpersonal climate of 12-step groups predicts reductions in alcohol use. *Alcoholism Treatment Quarterly, 31*(2), 167–185.

Smith, A. R. (2007). *The social world of Alcoholics Anonymous: How it works.* Lincoln, NE: iUniverse.

Walsh, J. (2013). *The recovery philosophy and direct social work practice.* Chicago, IL: Lyceum.

Yalom, I. D. (1970/1995). *The theory and practice of group psychotherapy* (4th ed.). New York, NY: Basic Books.

People with stigmatized conditions need a liberating meaning perspective that can free them from self-hate... and assumptions that they are inadequate.
BORKMAN (1999, p. 115)

8

ANALYZING A GROUP'S CLIMATE, PHILOSOPHY, AND STRUCTURE

YOU WALK INTO a room full of strangers, and you feel right at home. Why is that? People smile, sit quietly, look comfortable, and show interest in the program about to begin. Someone reads from a book that explains the group's philosophy and teachings. The group proceeds with the meeting in an orderly manner, and it is clear that someone has taken responsibility for making meetings go smoothly. There is no group leader, but regular members make sure that newcomers are introduced and the program is explained.

What you are about to experience is a group with a pleasant personality, a clear meaning perspective, and established structure. The group personality is called its social climate or group environment, a concept pioneered by Rudolf Moos (1981). The readings reveal how the group conveys its message—teachings about the condition and how to fix it. The smooth functioning of the meeting can also be attributed to how it is structured. The lack of professional intervention shows that the group has found a way to maintain a helping atmosphere without it. Each of these three issues—climate, philosophy, structure—will be explained here so they can be used for assessment and problem solving.

SOCIAL CLIMATE IN GROUPS

Social climate gives a group its unique personality by demonstrating high or low scores on ten dimensions called the Group Environment Scales (GES) (see box 8.1). The scales use standardized items, which makes it possible to compare the climate in your particular group with typical climates in other groups. These dimensions are measured by members' scores on either a paper or digital inventory. Informally, you can simply rate the group yourself after experiencing a typical meeting one or more times. Your rating of the group might help in figuring out why the group is struggling with something, such as lack of attendance or failure to self-disclose.

For example, participants in a new group for people with bipolar illness have met for three months with only sporadic attendance by most of the initial twelve attendees (except for the two leaders of the group, who also have bipolar conditions). In a meeting, members sit passively, waiting for the leaders to initiate conversation, and at one point, a participant expresses a wish to be educated by experts who are not fellow members. The group's founders had wanted it to be a support group wherein participants would share their experiential knowledge and methods of coping with mood swings, rather than have it be an educational forum dominated by professionals.

BOX 8.1
SUBSCALES OF THE GROUP ENVIRONMENT SCALE

- *Cohesion.* The commitment, concern, and friendship group members display for one another.
- *Leader support.* The amount of help, caring, and friendship the leader shows for group members.
- *Expressiveness.* The free expression of feelings encouraged by group members in meetings.
- *Independence.* How much the group encourages independent action and expression among members.
- *Task orientation.* How much emphasis is placed on completing concrete, practical tasks, decision-making, and training.
- *Independence.* How much the group encourages independent action and expression among members.
- *Discovery.* How much the group allows discussion of personal problems.
- *Anger and aggression.* How much open expression of anger and disagreement there is in the group.
- *Order and organization.* To what degree there are organization, structure, and rules in the group.
- *Leader control.* The extent to which the leader directs the group, makes decisions, and enforces rules.
- *Innovation.* How much the group promotes diversity and change.

Moos 1981. A license is required to use these scales in paper or digital format. Manual and scales are available at http://mindgarden.com/products/gescs.htm

Scrutiny of the interaction in this group's meetings would likely indicate that leader support was too low (new members did not receive as much help as they needed from the leaders). In terms of group environment, the leaders were not as task-oriented and expressive as members wanted; that is, they did not provide specific information and did not share personal stories that new members looked for to feel comfortable with them as role models. The leaders could attend to and alter these two dimensions and increase satisfaction with the group by sharing more about themselves. Or, bowing to the desire for outside input from experts, they could invite speakers with special knowledge as another way to bring their attendance up and meet member needs.

In the early 1990s, I asked self-help and support group members in groups for families of either mentally ill or addicted members to rate the climates in three separate groups: a local support group, an Al-Anon group, and a NAMI support group. They all rated their groups as very high in group cohesion, task orientation, and order and organization (Kurtz, 1992). They were extremely low in anger and aggression. The absence of a trained leader needs to be offset by a structured set of leader behaviors and meeting formats that are orderly and relatively task-oriented. Anger and aggression (defined as argumentative, confronting kinds of comments), in particular, need to be minimized, because participants need to feel safe from being criticized. This last advice is important in any group but especially so when newcomers are present. Box 8.2 gives a more detailed list of possible social climate interventions.

Using the GES, four AA groups were compared in an investigation of how the groups differed from one another (Montgomery, Miller, & Tonigan, 1993). At the time, AA groups were often discussed as if they were all alike, so the investigators wanted to assess the nature and degree of variation among groups. They used a modified version of the GES in which they removed items from the scales that did not apply to AA groups (leader control and task orientation). They also added items to reflect impressions of spirituality, the number of times the respondent had attended the group, and the number of months sober. What they found confirmed their hypothesis that AA groups do differ in some ways. They differed most on the cohesion and the anger and aggression subscales. The two groups that were less cohesive were higher in anger and aggression. This is not to suggest that the groups with higher anger and aggression engaged in physical confrontations, but members were more apt to disagree among themselves. This kind of assessment can be helpful in deciding where to refer new members and how to counsel them when discussing their participation.

BOX 8.2
CHANGING SOCIAL CLIMATE DIMENSIONS

Dimension	Facilitator Action
Higher cohesion	Increase homogeneity of members.
	Emphasize commonalities of members.
	Plan social events.
More leader support	Increase supportive comments.
	Move leader's chair closer to group.
Increased order/organization	Increase formal presentations.
	Use a meeting agenda.
	Develop standardized procedures.
Increased expressiveness	Use free-floating communication patterns.
Increased independence	Encourage expression and action in group.
Increased task orientation	Introduce structured exercises in meetings.
Increased leader control	Train leadership.
	Use an agenda in meetings.
Reduced anger/aggression	Verbalize ground rules and norms against it.
Increased innovation	Use less structure.
	Ask for new ideas.

GROUP PHILOSOPHY OR WORLDVIEW

In his book on self-help organizations for addictions, Keith Humphreys (2004, p. 128) pointed out that these associations are "more akin to communities than to treatments." These communities allow members to create an entire social circle in which they share friendship, attend social events, and develop an individual social network. This is particularly true of AA because of its large size and international spread, with groups in every small community and, in cities, in almost every neighborhood. In these settings, members encounter a philosophy and a set of values that Humphreys calls a "worldview." Others have termed these beliefs "ideologies," but this word has been contaminated by political discourse and no longer fits the subject being discussed here (Antze, 1979). A worldview involves beliefs about the problem and its cause, teachings that offer possible solutions and tools, and values concerning such things as spiritual beliefs in recovery.

Beliefs about the problem's causality lead to particular self-help methods. Overeaters Anonymous, for example, views overeating as a compulsion, similar to an addiction, and applies the twelve-step approach to it. A Weight Watchers group would view the problem more simply as a pattern of eating too much that can be corrected by sticking with a behavioral weight-loss program. It combines a complex method of attaching points to every bite of food intake, controlling that intake, with reporting in to a group or recording it online. In the group, efforts to follow the program get aired, and weights are taken; success is reinforced by group approval. But this is only one aspect of an organization's worldview. Members participate over time, and as their involvement deepens, the values and beliefs they acquire become more synchronized with the membership's values. These worldviews, acquired through lengthy and extensive involvement, have a greater impact on members' lives than might a briefer interval of professional treatment for an addiction-related or mental health condition. Members may participate in more than one chapter of the association, take part in social activities sponsored by them, work to keep the groups in existence, and make them a source of their friendship networks. Thus, this perspective applies well to the intense involvement of people in a recovering community composed of the dense networks of twelve-step fellowships. It may be less apropos for smaller, less complex support groups or newly emerging self-help associations than for larger organizations.

Borkman (1999) also saw the self-help association as a place where teachings and beliefs about the condition emerge from narratives within the group meetings. Based on her observations of a group for stutterers, she proposes a framework consisting of four components to capture the core teachings of a group, which she refers to as a "meaning perspective." The four components provide a means for gauging the group's understanding of the problem and its solution. Briefly, these are: (1) What is a useful way of defining the problem? (2) How do we define ourselves in relation to the problem and in a nonstigmatizing way? (3) How can we resolve the problem in a manner that is constructive, respectful, and dignified? (4) How do we organize our collective and our relationships with ourselves and others in our problem solving and recovery? As Borkman pointed out, a group's meaning perspective takes a while to develop, so a group may be in a fledgling stage in which its frame is just beginning to evolve, or it may have taken on the more mature framework, such as that of twelve-step groups, without having yet gained the maturity as a group to understand it fully. You can assess your group's philosophy or teachings by using Borkman's framework as presented in box 8.3.

Member stories are a major way in which the group's philosophy and program are communicated to new participants and to others. In twelve-step fellowships, the story is told in three parts: what it was like (with the problem), what happened (the

BOX 8.3
FRAMEWORK FOR IDENTIFYING CORE TEACHINGS OF A GROUP

Condition defined	Out-of-control drinker (eater, etc.)
Nonstigmatizing identity	Recovering alcoholic (overeater)
Constructive resolution	Going to meetings, sharing stories, following the steps, service to others
How group is structured	Small groups or speaker meetings, sharing stories of recovery

Borkman (1999).

crisis that turned things around), and what it's like now (in the fellowship of recovery). Other self-help organizations have similar ways of structuring a story that conveys how the association's program works. Paul's story (box 8.4) gives an example of how he used these tools in Recovery International.

In Paul's story, you see that the condition is defined as "social anxiety." The nonstigmatizing identity in Recovery International parlance would be "nervousness around people." The constructive resolution is "attending Recovery meetings, reading the literature, and practicing the method." The group is structured around "voluntary panel presentations by participants in meetings," where they give examples of their spotting and practice of methods. Any group should strive to identify itself within each of the four parts of the framework so as to articulate the group's core teachings. Most self-help fellowships and organizations have these elements, although they may need to be enunciated more clearly for participants.

GROUP STRUCTURE

A group's structure involves its size, meeting format, leadership positions, rules, regulations, and procedures. Many self-help groups belong to large national associations that contribute structure, such as by giving affiliated groups a meeting format to follow and recommending leadership positions. Self-help organizations should seek not to become bureaucracies but only to have the basic structure to function smoothly and apply methods and meeting procedures. As Borkman (1999, p. 167) noted, "the idea of a hierarchical organization [is] a knee-jerk reaction" in our society. Self-help and support groups should try to avoid too much structure.

BOX 8.4
PAUL'S STORY

My problem all my life has been social anxiety. It began when I was six or seven years old. I was very sensitive to criticism and would get upset when I made minor mistakes. I had almost no social life at all between the ages of eleven and thirty-two, because I felt so uncomfortable with people, and it seemed I didn't know how to start a conversation or make friends. I spent my free time reading books and watching television. In the meantime, I had psychotherapy for several years with a psychoanalyst, which helped me quite a bit and got me feeling somewhat more relaxed with people, but I still couldn't make friends. After a few years, the therapist said I had reached a "plateau" and didn't seem to be improving any further, so we broke off the sessions.

I met my future wife, Mary, when I was thirty-two years old. She asked me out on our first date; otherwise, I never would have had the nerve to approach her. She and I hit it off, and I felt more comfortable with her than I had with other people. We were married after dating for a year. She had nervous problems herself and had been going to Recovery International meetings (at that time, it was called Recovery, Inc.), and she recommended it to me. I started going to the meetings from time to time, but it wasn't until sometime in 1989 that I realized that the Recovery method was the thing that could really help me get better and that I needed to study the literature, attend meetings every week, and practice the method. One thing that happened after a few weeks of attending regularly is that I made a mistake bringing my laundry in to the cleaners, and I began to get very upset. I told myself that my uncomfortable feelings were distressing but not dangerous, and I realized that there was no reason to blame myself for my mistake, because it was an average mistake, and it was just a triviality of everyday life. The upset feelings faded within minutes.

Since then, I've been attending meetings regularly and practicing the method. I began leading a Recovery meeting in 1995, which I never could have done before. I find that Recovery training combines well with psychotherapy sessions with my psychiatrist. My social anxiety and fear of making mistakes have gradually decreased. I feel comfortable with people like I never did before, I'm able to joke and make conversation with strangers, and I don't get upset when I make a mistake or receive criticism nearly as much as I did. I apply the Recovery methods of spotting and muscle control many times each day to deal with the everyday trivialities that maintain nervous symptoms. That has made my life much better than it was before I found out about Recovery International.

These groups tend to be open-ended; that is, they do not limit the number of members, and anyone who qualifies can join. This makes the size flexible and could result in large groups. Other groups' memberships are controlled by the organization that sponsors them. For example, a local hospital may offer a support group for families but limit it to the families it specifically refers. Another hospital may list a support group for families on its website and invite anyone from the local community to attend. It's always understood that participants must fit the definition of one who has the identity of those served by the group; for instance, a group for families of alcoholics should be limited to them and not open to anyone else who is interested. The reason for this is straightforward. The group helps by having members share experiential knowledge about the one issue they have in common; those without that one issue will derive little and will not offer anything for the rest of the group to use.

Groups typically structure their meetings along the following lines: assigning door greeters to welcome newcomers and regular members, serving refreshments that encourage informal mingling before meetings, beginning meetings with an introductory reading that explains the group's purpose, establishing a set pattern of sharing stories, and arranging the room in a certain way, such as seating people in a circle. There should usually be someone in charge of the meeting, even if the group is philosophically opposed to having a hierarchy. The leadership role can rotate. People should introduce themselves unless everyone knows one another. There should be an established pattern for speaking up in meetings so that everyone who wants to talk has a chance to do so.

Usually, problems that can be traced to structure reflect lack of it. When there are no roles for regular members, newer people may feel confused, uncertain, or left out altogether. Some people may talk too much, dominate the group's meeting, and fail to include new members in the discussion. People may be unclear about the group's purpose and irritated by its disorganization. Lack of leadership positions that split the duties involved in running the organization may lead to things being left undone or some people being overburdened by taking on too much of the work. One of the easiest fixes for groups that flounder is to add structure.

Just having a leader will lend necessary structure to some groups. A designated leader can correct any problems with structure that interfere with the meeting's process. This person can appoint a member to play the role of greeter, whose mission is to make members feel welcome. A leader can arrange the chairs in a circle and introduce some reading of group literature or the group's mission statement at the beginning of the meeting. New members may introduce themselves. It might work to have regular members say their names and share something about why they are in the group. This can be achieved by going around the circle. After this is completed, there should be some time left to open the meeting for discussion of specific issues. These may involve problems, or they may, even better, involve progress. The leader can ask the speaker to tell how he or she accomplished something positive. The leader can end the meeting with some form of closure, such as the Serenity Prayer in a twelve-step meeting. This is structure.

You have accomplished making people feel welcome. You have let each member know why the group meets and what it hopes to accomplish. You have let each person know that everyone shares the same problem identity. You have entertained spoken examples of progress by older members, which give newcomers hope, one of the key factors in recovery.

TWELVE-STEP MEETING STRUCTURE

For readers unfamiliar with the structure and process of a typical twelve-step meeting, this description offers some generalizations, mindful that such groups are autonomous and can change procedures to suit the situation or the makeup of a particular group. Most twelve-step groups use a printed meeting agenda for leaders to follow. These leaders rotate into the role for a limited period of time, but this is not a position of authority, and so they are not free to change the usual meeting routine. Although there are other twelve-step groups, what follows describes varieties of an Alcoholics Anonymous meeting.

After any necessary preliminary announcements, every meeting itself begins with a prayer, usually the Serenity Prayer, and a reading from the "Big Book" (1976). The reading typically comes from chapter 5, "How It Works" (pp. 58–60), which includes the twelve steps. There are several types of meetings, such as discussion, speaker, Big Book study, and step meetings. Large groups that hold discussion meetings typically break into small groups for discussion after the preliminary reading. After a topic is chosen, discussion may follow a go-around pattern in which each person may comment. Alternatively, participants may speak randomly though only once. This gives everyone the opportunity to speak but also allows an individual to say, "I am just listening today." Although reference may be made to another person's "share," the norm within this discussion is "no crosstalk," a practice adopted by the earliest AAs in reaction against the Oxford Group practice of "Guidance," in which members often told others what to do (Ernest Kurtz, personal communication, April 15, 2014).

Speaker meetings begin with the Serenity Prayer and a Big Book reading, after which the chosen speaker comes to the podium and tells his or her story, following the pattern described under the discussion of philosophy. The speaker is not interrupted, and the presentation is usually followed by a break for coffee and perhaps other refreshments. Participants then regather briefly for any announcements and often continue to chat about the presentation. Newcomers do not give their stories (often called leads), because their stories are not complete until they begin to identify with other members and have some success in using the program.

Two important notes: Nonmembers sometimes refer to member stories as "catharsis," but this is incorrect. A catharsis is a relief of emotional tension. The twelve-step story is the main way the program is conveyed among members, by showing how it works. People also sometimes call a story a "drunkalog." If the story contains only the first part, or "what it was like," then it is a drunkalog—it tells only of being drunk. This sometimes happens when a speaker enjoys describing the humorous antics of his or her drinking days—when this part of the story goes disproportionately long, it becomes a drunkalog. A well-formed story with all three parts is not a drunkalog.

Big Book study and step meetings are what their names imply. After the preliminary announcements, prayer, and reading, a chapter or other segment of the Big Book AA, 1939/1976) or a step in the book *The Twelve Steps and Twelve Traditions* (AA, 1953) is read, and then members break into small groups to discuss the reading. The practice in these groups follows what has been described for discussion meetings.

CONCLUSION

This chapter highlighted some of the concepts you can apply to understanding your meeting as a group and how some common problems can be addressed using group environment assessments, articulating a philosophy or worldview, or changing structural elements. There is no one right way to lead a group, but there are aspects of groups that can be measured or characterized for better understanding of their functioning and for setting goals. The ideas presented here will not solve every problem you encounter. Some challenges in your group may have more to do with specific members, the stage of recovery they are in, or members' personality differences. The next chapter will cover aspects of individual members and some of the factors that influence their participation in a group, such as change-readiness, stage of affiliation, and characteristics of long-term members.

REFERENCES

AA. (1939/1976). *Alcoholics Anonymous: The story of how many thousands of men and women have recovered from alcoholism* (3rd ed.). New York, NY: AA World Services.

AA. (1953). *The Twelve Steps and Twelve Traditions.* New York, NY: AA World Services.

Antze, P. A. (1979). The role of ideologies in peer psychotherapy groups. In M. A. Lieberman and L. Borman (Eds.), *Self-help groups for coping with crisis* (pp. 272–304). San Francisco, CA: Jossey-Bass.

Borkman, T. J. (1999). *Understanding self-help/mutual aid: Experiential learning in the commons.* New Brunswick, NJ: Rutgers University Press.

Humphreys, K. (2004). *Circles of recovery: Self-help organizations for addictions.* Cambridge: Cambridge University Press.

Kurtz, L. F. (1992). Group environments in self-help groups for families. *Small Group Research, 23*, 199–215.

Montgomery, H. A., Miller, W. R., & Tonigan, J. S. (1993). Differences among AA groups: Implications for research. *Journal of Studies on Alcohol, 54*, 502–504.

Moos, R. H. (1981). *Group Environment Scale manual.* Menlo Park, CA: Mind Garden.

[T]he investigation of any trait in alcoholics will show they have either more or less of it.
KELLER (1972, p. 1147)

9

WHO NEEDS A GROUP? THE PROCESS OF AFFILIATION

DAVID RUDY, SOCIOLOGIST and college professor, sat in his car outside the church where an AA group was about to begin its meeting. Having arrived twenty minutes early, Rudy was nervous. He thought about his entry into an open meeting where he hoped to gather data for his participant observation study of the AA fellowship. Questions raced through his mind. Would he be asked to leave? Would he know anyone there? What if no one wanted to talk to him? He needn't have worried. The group accepted him, and when he continued to go to meetings, they began to think of him as an alcoholic. They couldn't imagine someone attending that many meetings for sixteen months without having some reason other than research. His research culminated in the book *Becoming Alcoholic: Alcoholics Anonymous and the Reality of Alcoholism*, published in 1986. Rudy wanted to know how people became attached to the fellowship and how they constructed an alcoholic identity. His findings and interpretation will be summarized later in this chapter.

Without new members, recovery groups die, and without group involvement, most participants relapse (Bond, Kaskutas, & Weisner, 2003; Vaillant, 2003; Wituk, Shepherd, Warren, & Meissen, 2002). This makes the questions of who joins, who stays, and why critical. At least 40 percent of those referred to a recovery group after treatment drop out in early stages (Kelly & Moos, 2003). By identifying the features of successful and unsuccessful linkage with groups, we can predict who may need extra supports to make the transition from hesitant beginning to regular, reliable participation. Rudy's interest was in the processes involved in becoming an AA member. Earlier and later research has looked instead at the background characteristics of AA members. Before discussing Rudy's findings, let's consider some of those characteristics.

WHO COMES BACK

Several early investigations on characteristics of AA members found that they tended to be middle-class socioeconomically, especially those who succeeded and remained active for longer periods (Boscarino, 1980; Rudy, 1986). In the past, researchers thought that middle-class people were more likely to affiliate with a group that required reading literature, finding and attending meetings, and participating in a verbal, problem-sharing activity, which included speaking before a group at times. Two studies going back the 1950s and '60s examined AA receptivity to newcomers of working-class status (Lofland & Lejeune, 1960; Murphy, 1953). Both found members in groups they observed to be open to newcomers regardless of class, appearance, and behavior.

Problem seriousness also distinguishes those who attach to a recovery group. The idea of hitting bottom has remained an important indicator of openness to getting help, even though some say it should not be (Tonigan, Bogenschutz, & Miller, 2006). Persons who report losing control of their drinking, consuming a higher quantity of alcohol when drinking, and drinking compulsively are more likely to continue with and benefit from recovery group participation (Emrick, Tonigan, Montgomery, & Little, 1993). Psychological distress correlates with involvement in almost any recovery group, whether it is for physical illness such as cancer, mental illness, or substance disorder (Davison, Pennebaker, & Dickerson, 2000; Humphreys, Mavis, & Stofflemayr, 1995; Kurtz, 1997; Maton, 1988).

Being an Extrovert and Need for Affiliation

Being extroverted and having a high need for affiliation with others have come up often in efforts to identify who succeeds in a recovery self-help/support group. In Harrison Trice's early study of affiliation with AA (1957), he found that having a self-conception of being a person who could share basic emotional reactions with others was more meaningful as a predictor of later affiliation than feeling "licked" (problem seriousness) or labeling oneself an alcoholic. Trice (1959) later called willingness to share the affiliation motive. He identified three phases of affiliation: before going to any meeting, time of initial contact with a group, and after attending meetings for a few weeks. His formulations and research into this concept now seem way ahead of his time. Understanding the affiliation process gives us a different way of looking at linking members with the fellowship. Although characteristics of successful and unsuccessful recruits give some understanding of eventual affiliation, knowing what stage of affiliation someone is in provides additional help in knowing how to link people with groups.

Openness to Spirituality

Openness to spirituality is another characteristic that could predict whether individuals remain attached to AA or other twelve-step groups that have a spiritual component (Emrick et al., 1993; Kelly & Moos, 2003; Krentzman, Robinson, Perron, & Cranford, 2011). Openness to the concept of God, experience of religion in childhood, and former participation in religious activity predispose people to affiliate with AA. Researchers examining whether spiritual and religious changes in a twelve-step program affected later progress found a positive outcome in drinking behavior in those whose spirituality and openness to religion had increased through their participation (Robinson, Krentzman, Webb, & Brower, 2011).

The religious tone and deliberate spiritual connotations of twelve-step fellowships have driven many potential recruits away from them and resulted in a number of secular groups, such as LifeRing, Secular Organization for Sobriety, and AA Agnostica (Roger C., 2014). It is likely that the spiritual component in the large AA and NA networks has both attracted and repelled thousands of potential members. Secular groups have struggled to find an effective hold on members while trying, sometimes unsuccessfully, to respect their spiritually oriented competitors. Their rise in recent years has given many addicts an alternative to twelve-step recovery. The controversies about spirituality in recovery have not stretched to recovery groups for other conditions. GROW and Schizophrenics Anonymous have mild spiritual components; Recovery International does not have any. Secular substitutes for Emotions Anonymous and Overeaters Anonymous do not exist.

The Importance of Group Fit

There is a tendency for newcomers and outsiders to look at one group in an extensive network, such as AA, and then assume that all AA groups are the same. An apocryphal story is of the researcher who went to one meeting of AA that had a coffee pot in the middle of the table. He wrote in his report that AA groups all meet with coffee pots on the table. In fact, groups take on the characteristics of the local community or any number of other factors, and this makes each group unique. Groups with a majority of people of a particular race, gender, or sexual orientation have grown that way as a result of something called person-group fit (Luke, Roberts, & Rappaport, 1993; Kelly & Moos, 2003). For example, a group of older white men will be attractive to other older white men, and newcomers not fitting that identity, while welcome, may go elsewhere where they fit in better. In a large city, among AA groups, because there are so many, it is possible to find a group in which one fits by gender, age, race, or other demographics and also by personal philosophy, such as belief in a higher power.

Race, gender, and sexual orientation may vary by group and by where the groups meet. When I was doing research for my dissertation in the state of Georgia, I met and interviewed one very tall, thin, eighty-two-year-old African American man. He told me about his addictions, everything from moonshine to laudanum; he had been drinking for fifty-nine years when he became ill and near death; he languished in a coma for four months. Upon recovery, he went to his first AA meeting, prompted by fear of what would happen if he drank again. The group met at the state hospital. He told of how he opened the door to the meeting room, where ten or fifteen white men and women sat in a circle. At first, there was complete silence as this very dark-skinned man stood looking in, almost ready to flee. Finally, a man in the circle said, "Come on in here and sit down; you're one of us." He went in, stayed sober, and had been a member for nine years when I met him in 1982. The fact of his participation led many more African American alcoholics to the fellowship in that central Georgia town of Milledgeville in the 1970s and '80s. It was unusual that this black man was willing to enter an all-white group in the deep South in 1973 and not drop out.

Similarly, Marty Mann, the first woman in AA, was admitted to the all-male New York group in the organization's early years despite some initial controversy. Now approximately 35 percent of AA's membership is female (AA, 2013). Except for AA, NA, and Gamblers Anonymous, however, most self-help and support group memberships are predominantly female. NA's membership is close to 50 percent female (47 percent).

The issue of group fit cannot be underestimated as an element of concern when linking people to addiction and mental health recovery groups. While it may not be possible to locate a group that matches a consumer's age, race, gender, and social class, this can be a topic to explore with the individual being connected to a group. For gregarious people who enjoy group participation, simply discussing these issues may be enough to allay concerns. For more introverted or shy people, Annette Smith's (2007) qualitative study of AA revealed a process for linking people with low needs for affiliation and group dependency to the fellowship (see figure 9.1). Her research on this subject found that people who were less group-oriented than the extroverts did affiliate but did so in a slightly different way. In addition, some did so because they could not stay sober any other way.

As the figure shows, linking a potential recruit to an individual member is preferable to sending someone to a group alone (see chapter 5). The helping person (temporary sponsor) can get to know the recruit and take him or her to a meeting, or to several meetings, until the newcomer indicates a willingness to go alone. There should be follow-up by the sponsor to be sure the recruit actually goes. Many people resist participation because they sense that they will be

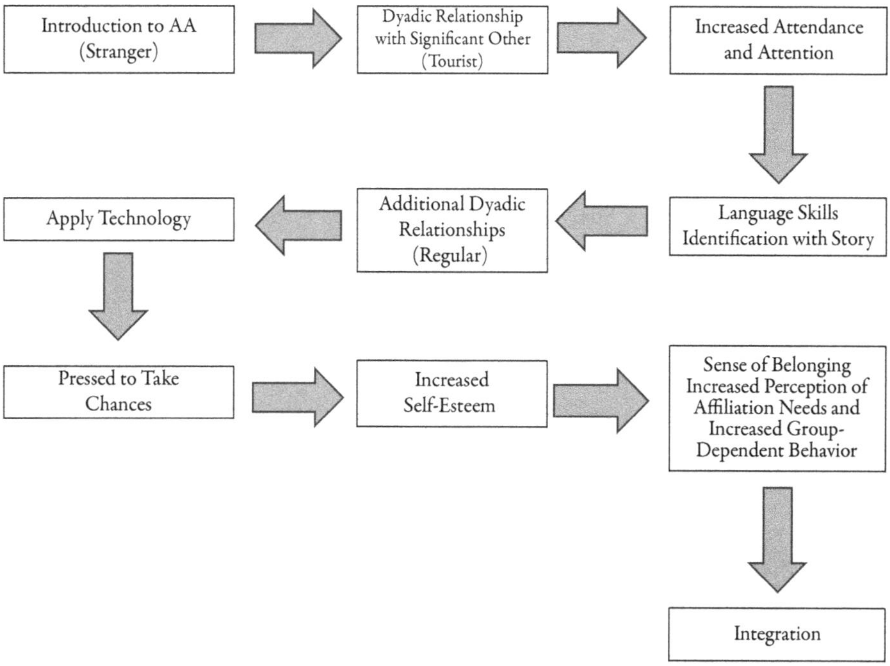

FIGURE 9.1 AA Integration of Persons with Low Degree of Affiliation Need
From Smith (2007). Used with permission.

encouraged to talk in the group. New recruits should be assured that they can pass, and all they have to say is "I pass" when the group go-around gets to them. Eventually, they may be asked to speak up in the group, but they will not be forced to do so. Before or after the meetings, newcomers will meet other individuals with whom they can share information about themselves, and they will gradually become affiliated with one or more local groups, and one will become their home group.

AFFILIATION AS A PROCESS

The affiliation process has been examined by numerous authors of research on various types of groups (Jurik, 1987; Raiff, 1979; Klass, 1984–85; Rudy 1986; Smith, 2007; Trice, 1957). Another stagelike theory that predicts affiliation constancy is that of readiness to change (DiClemente, 1993). These approaches are similar in that they look at the evolution of an individual's efforts to use the recovery community as a means of making a life change. For addicts, the change involves not using a substance, which also means giving up the relationships they have with others who use and facing up to problems that the substance has covered up. For people with emotional problems, it means associating with a new set of people and possibly also changing in other ways. This is not just a matter of not drinking, not drugging, or not giving in to psychiatric symptoms. It is commitment to a different way of life.

Studies of recovery groups for mental health and of AA have noted that inductees go through stages in their participation levels, ending with successful integration into the organization. Jurik (1987), in her ethnographic study of Recovery International (Recovery, Inc., at the time), thought of the stages she observed as a persuasion process. The first stage in this process consisted of the first five meetings, in which the new recruit is encouraged to participate, and older members explain how the group has helped them. They encourage the recruit to see the first meeting as a turning point. The second phase involves the new recruit's understanding of the problem, so it conforms to the psychiatric framework taught by Recovery, which locates its source in one's own personality rather than in social injustice or religious sources. Further, Abraham Low believed that the condition was not related to past events or present environment but is located in the member's reactions to situations, reactions that can be modified by using the Recovery program. The next phase entailed the implementation of Recovery techniques in daily encounters and reported on progress in meetings by giving panel examples. In the fourth stage, the member presents panel examples skillfully and approaches new recruits.

Rudy's research identified six phases in the process of affiliation with AA (see table 9.1). He found that the process started earlier than Jurik's beginning stage in Recovery, Inc. Rudy called the first phase "hitting bottom." This is the stage in which the alcoholic realizes that his or her condition is not going away and is not amenable to individual efforts of willpower and that the situation has become intolerable. Sometimes a period of treatment intervenes, but that has seldom been enough to stop the alcoholic's downward path. Hitting bottom often requires that the individual be forced through confrontation to recognize the necessity of getting help and going to that first meeting.

The second stage, "first-stepping," involves making the initial contact with AA. At this point, the recruit has been connected to a group and has attended a meeting. He or she learns that the only requirement for membership is a desire to stop drinking; if the recruit wants to stop drinking, he or she qualifies. Newcomers are encouraged to listen rather than talk. Newcomers hear others' stories and realize that they are similar to their own—they identify. AA's primary purpose is to help the alcoholic who still suffers; therefore, members go out of their way to be warm and accepting of newcomers, to help them realize that they belong in AA. The greeting given to the elderly black man in Milledgeville, Georgia—"Come on in here and sit down; you are one of us"—exemplifies this "open arms" approach to newcomers. The overarching goal of "carrying the message" sinks in with new members quickly and overshadows reservations about personal qualities such as race, gender, or sexual orientation.

TABLE 9.1
PROCESS OF AFFILIATION WITH AA

Hitting bottom	New recruit is forced to realize that he or she has reached the point of needing to stop using or drinking; a crisis or turning point.
First-stepping	Making an initial contact with the group/program; received warmly by members.
Making a commitment	When ready, newcomer is pressured to devote time to the program, possibly 90 meetings in 90 days, and to read and understand the program's literature.
Accepting one's problem	The recruit begins to accept the identity of being an alcoholic (addict, etc.).
Telling one's story	Most members tell their story of what it was like (before program), what happened, and what it's like now (since joining), usually within six months of first contact.
Doing twelve-step work	Member "carries the message" to the alcoholic who still suffers. Helping others is what keeps the member sober.

Rudy (1986).

"Making a commitment" comes next, once the recruit has shown interest by attending several meetings. Old-timers pressure the recruit to make a behavioral commitment by taking on small tasks for the group, such as coming early and setting up the meeting room or making coffee. These small tasks are a way to give newcomers with low bottoms (those who have lost jobs, family, homes) a sense of responsibility and belonging. Attendance is also rewarded with engraved poker chips or coins in various colors representing time sober, along with acknowledgment and applause in the home group. Newcomers at this stage are often asked to commit to "90/90" (ninety meetings in ninety days). This has the effect of removing the temptations to go back to the old lifestyle with drinking friends. Close relatives may attend Al-Anon or Nar-Anon. Old-timers encourage newcomers to get sponsors and to hang out with program members at places such as Alano Clubs (private clubs run by members), where meetings go on throughout the day and members can sit around and talk; other AA groups sometimes recruit workers for businesses they own or for other work.

Rudy calls the fourth phase "accepting one's problem." New recruits begin AA attendance before they really accept their problem as alcoholism. This is one reason they drop out early in their participation—not really believing they truly have the condition. Regular members talk about how dropouts need to do more research—the research being trying a few more times to drink socially without getting drunk. This stage is one of identity transformation, realizing that they cannot succeed at social drinking and that the problem is real. The recruit begins to apply the program seriously, finding a sponsor, taking a moral inventory (fourth step), and sharing it with someone else (fifth step).

The fifth phase consists of "telling one's story." The story requires that the teller be able to say how things were before getting sober or clean, what happened to stop the drinking or using, and how things are now that the storyteller has been sober (clean) in the twelve-step program. It requires that the storyteller have a period of sobriety in the fellowship so that the story ends on a positive note and is not just a drunkalog. Rudy likens this to a commitment act symbolizing the initiate's incorporation into the group, usually expected at six months.

The final phase of the affiliation process is "carrying the message"; in twelve-step programs, this is twelfth-step work. Members reach out to those who need help as a way of renewing their realization that they are just one drink away from being in the same boat. Helping others is a way of threefold helping: the other, oneself, and the fellowship. This is central to the idea that recovery communities need older, experienced members if they are to remain effective.

Rudy concludes his description of the six phases by suggesting that he has discovered why some drop out and others remain involved. Instead of asking if affiliates have certain characteristics, we should ask about what happened when the affiliate moved through the phases. Did crucial events occur? Did the recruit go willingly to the first group, or was it forced on him or her? Did the potential member know others who supported the idea of membership, or did he or she receive opposition from people important to him or her? Did the recruit observe others in initial meetings with whom he or she identified? These factors are essential to encouraging attachment at different points. Pushing a brand-new member to get up and tell his or her story, for example, would be counterproductive and probably scare the person away. For one thing, this person would not have a story of recovery to tell because he or she had not yet experienced the payoff of being sober long enough.

The recognition that member affiliation in a group like AA, or many other recovery groups, is a process that comes over time and needs to be prodded along in different ways is not a new one, and it gets rediscovered periodically by those interested in addiction recovery. It is not, however, as well recognized with regard to other recovery groups, such as Recovery International or membership in a clubhouse. Change-readiness, however, is something that can apply to any group or treatment program.

STAGES OF CHANGE-READINESS

A conceptualization based on research that applies more broadly to people in recovery is the "transtheoretical model of change," which began with research on recovery from nicotine addiction but can be applied to any situation or anyone who faces a demand for change (DiClemente, 1993). The stages outlined in that model correspond to the stages in the affiliation process that we have just discussed (see table 9.2). The stages of change-readiness begin with the precontemplation stage, in which individuals are not interested in changing even though others think they should, which is similar to the hitting bottom stage. The next stage is contemplation, recognizing the need for change and giving it serious consideration. This would be parallel to the first-stepping phase of affiliation in which the recruit attends some meetings without making a commitment. The next stage of change-readiness is preparation, in which the individual makes a decision to change and begins a plan of action. These three beginning stages lead to the action stage, where efforts to make the change are most obvious while the individual carries out his or her plan. If successful, the individual enters a maintenance stage, where the task is to sustain the behavior change in the future. Anyone who has ever lost weight can identify with the importance of the maintenance stage. It is here that relapses happen: someone takes one drink that leads to many more, someone gives in to episodes of temper that lead to a breakdown, or someone eats that whole cheesecake and cannot stop.

PROCESSES OF CHANGE

Certain processes of change are appropriate to each of the stages of change. For example, consciousness raising is a process that occurs in the precontemplation stage, before the individual realizes that a problem exists or how serious it is. DiClemente (1993) observes that exposing a new recruit to the recovery group's message and taking a tolerant attitude that allows the unconvinced novice the latitude to continue experiencing the negative effects of the behavior is the best way to get precontemplators to take the first step. He points out that recovery group principles and practices are not designed to reach precontemplators, because they assume that the person attending meetings has reached a taking-action stage much sooner than it is reasonable to expect. Precontemplators react negatively to spiritual messages about a higher power, pressure for total abstinence (one day at a time), and labeling oneself an alcoholic. They have to be convinced, and some never submit to that message.

Recovery group activities are well adapted to the person who is beginning to consider a change at the contemplation stage. The contemplator recognizes the activities required of him or her in order to continue in the fellowship, such as attending

TABLE 9.2
PHASES OF AFFILIATION, LEVELS OF CHANGE, AND HOW CHANGE IS ADDRESSED IN TWELVE-STEP FELLOWSHIPS

Stage of Affiliation	Level of Change-Readiness	Processes That Support Change
Hitting bottom	Precontemplation—individual sees no problem.	Consciousness raising about the need to change; exposure to the group and message of hope works best at this stage.
First-stepping	Contemplation—willing to consider what is required to change.	Listening to member stories and identifying with speakers.
Making a commitment	Preparation—forming a plan of action.	Member pushed to take on tasks, attend 90 meetings in 90 days, receives recognition for milestones.
Accepting one's problem	Action—taking action.	Member can say "I'm an alcoholic" and mean it; identity transformation. Meeting participation, support from sponsor, performs twelve-step work, moves away from an alcoholic (drug-taking) lifestyle.
Telling one's story	Action.	Constructing a story in which the member confirms an alcoholic (drug-taking, etc.) identity and acknowledging the change taking place. Receives recognition from group.
Twelve-step work	Maintenance—AA offers a support system for building recovery capital to sustain change.	Carrying the message to others (twelfth-stepping), continuing participation, sponsoring others.

DiClemente (1993).

frequent meetings, abstaining from use, and getting a sponsor. DiClemente states, however, that helping persons may become impatient with contemplators who have not yet stopped the problem behavior (drinking, drugging, overeating, etc.), but contemplation without immediate action is a typical stage in the change process. It is important to recognize that the new recruit is headed for change and to sustain his or her contact with the group.

For individuals who have made a decision to stop using, recovery group principles and action steps offer obvious avenues for forming a plan for change in the preparation stage. For those in twelve-step groups, choosing a sponsor, taking inventory, listing persons harmed, attending meetings, and making amends are just some of the activities available for planned action. These activities are carried out in the action stage, along with social events, reading literature, and talking to a sponsor, if one is in a twelve-step program. The more groups and meetings available, the more one can reinforce the decision to change by substituting an entirely new way of life for the old one.

The maintenance stage within a recovery group goes on indefinitely for some people in recovery. These are the people who construct the social world of the recovery program for others and keep it going. Some academics and researchers from outside the fellowship see the never-ending nature of this form of recovery as a problem. DiClemente (1993, p. 92), for example, writes that there are "indications that continued self-re-evaluation long into action and maintenance can contribute to relapse rather than protect against it. There is no clear message as to when individuals can disengage from meetings." Others would regard the committed, longtime members as insiders within the social world of AA or another recovery program (Smith, 2007). Insiders' focus is on making sure that the program activities continue and that newcomers receive an immediate response to their efforts to get help. Without insiders, the fellowship could be in danger of failing in its purpose. Their participation has become a way of life, with challenges, social relationships, and high points. Often family members either join them as fellow recovering members or as members of Al-Anon or Alateen.

CONCLUSION

There are characteristics that can predict how well certain individuals respond to a recovery group such as AA. Some of them are particular to AA and other twelve-step programs, such as openness to spirituality, and others are more general, such as being comfortable talking about problems in groups and being an extroverted person. The notion of group fit suggests that people will gravitate toward groups in which they see themselves fitting in, particularly with regard to race, ethnicity, and gender. Another way of thinking about linking individuals to a recovery group is to consider the typical stages of affiliation and anticipate what kind of support a person needs. This fits in with the concept of stages of change-readiness.

A new recruit may need to "do more research" (i.e., more drinking or drugging) before being ready to commit himself or herself to participation in a recovery group. Stages of change-readiness fit closely with the affiliation phases, in which the person begins in a precontemplation stage, not thinking about changing or not having hit bottom. At each stage, there are appropriate approaches to helping someone attach to the group.

The next chapter contains lengthy descriptions of some of the more well-known and larger recovery organizations in the United States. These include Al-Anon Family Groups, Recovery International, Schizophrenics Anonymous, and Dual Recovery Anonymous. These descriptions will show how a group other than the original AA, Al-Anon Family Groups, adapts and uses the twelve-step program; how another group, Recovery International, uses an entirely different set of concepts for establishing recovery; how Schizophrenics Anonymous has taken the twelve-step pattern and made it a six-step program; and how Dual Recovery Anonymous has rewritten the steps and traditions to conform to its needs for addressing both mental health conditions and addictions.

REFERENCES

AA. (2013). *Alcoholics Anonymous: 2011 Membership Survey.* Retrieved from www.aa.org

Bond, J., Kaskutas, L. A., & Weisner, C. (2003). The persistent influence of social networks and Alcoholics Anonymous on abstinence. *Journal of Studies on Alcohol, 64*(4), 579–588.

Boscarino, J. (1980). Factors related to "stable" and "unstable" affiliation with Alcoholics Anonymous. *International Journal of the Addictions, 15*(6), 839–848.

Davison, K. P., Pennebaker, J. W., & Dickerson, S. S. (2000).Who talks? The social psychology of illness support groups. *American Psychologist, 55*(2), 205–217.

DiClemente, C. C. (1993). Alcoholics Anonymous and the structure of change. In B. S. McCrady & W. R. Miller (Eds.), *Research on Alcoholics Anonymous: Opportunities and alternatives* (pp. 79–98). New Brunswick, NJ: Rutgers Center on Alcohol Studies.

Emrick, C., Tonigan, J. S., Montgomery, H. A., & Little, L. (1993). Alcoholics Anonymous: What is currently known. In B. S. McCrady & W. R. Miller (Eds.), *Research on Alcoholics Anonymous: Opportunities and alternatives* (pp. 41–76). New Brunswick, NJ: Rutgers Center on Alcohol Studies.

Humphreys, K., Mavis, B., & Stofflemayr, B. (1995). Are twelve step programs appropriate for disenfranchised groups? Evidence from a study of post-treatment involvement. In F. Lavoie, T. Borkman, & B. Gidron (Eds.), *Self-help and mutual aid groups: International and multicultural perspectives* (pp. 165–179). New York, NY: Haworth.

Jurik, N. C. (1987). Persuasion in a self-help group: Processes and consequences. *Small Group Behavior, 18*(3), 368–397.

Keller, M. (1972). The oddities of alcoholics. *Quarterly Journal of Studies on Alcohol, 33*(4), 1147–1148.

Kelly, J. F., & Moos, R. (2003). Dropout from 12-step self-help groups: Prevalence, predictors, and counteracting treatment influences. *Journal of Substance Abuse Treatment, 24*, 241–250.

Klass, D. (1984–1985). Bereaved parents and the Compassionate Friends: Affiliation and healing. *Omega Journal of Death and Dying, 15*, 353–373.

Krentzman, A. R., Robinson, E. A. R., Perron, B. E., & Cranford, J. A. (2011). Predictors of membership in Alcoholics Anonymous, in a sample of successfully remitted alcoholics. *Journal of Psychoactive Drugs, 43*(1), 20–26.

Kurtz, L. F. (1997). *Self-help and support groups: A handbook for practitioners.* Thousand Oaks, CA: Sage.

Lofland, J., & Lejeune, R. (1960). Initial interaction of newcomers in Alcoholics Anonymous. *Social Problems, 8*, 102–111.

Luke, D. A., Roberts, L., & Rappaport, J. (1993). Individual, group context, and individual-group fit predictors of self-help-group attendance. *Journal of Applied Behavioral Science, 29*, 216–238.

Maton, K. I. (1988). Social support, organizational characteristics, psychological well being, and group appraisal in three self-help group populations. *American Journal of Community Psychology, 16*(1), 203–232.

Murphy, M. M. (1953). Values stressed by two social class levels at meetings of Alcoholics Anonymous. *Quarterly Journal of Studies on Alcohol, 14*(4), 577–585.

Raiff, N. R. (1979). *Recovery, Inc.: A study of a self-help organization in mental health* (Unpublished doctoral dissertation). University of Pittsburgh, Pittsburgh, PA.

Robinson, E. A. R., Krentzman, A. R., Webb, J. R., & Brower, K. J. (2011). Six-month changes in spirituality and religiousness in alcoholics predict drinking outcomes at nine months. *Journal of Studies on Alcohol and Drugs, 72*(4), 660–688.

Roger C. (Ed.). (2014). *Don't tell: Stories and essays by agnostics and atheists in AA.* Toronto, ON: AA Agnostica.

Rudy, D. R. (1986). *Becoming alcoholic: Alcoholics Anonymous and the reality of alcoholism.* Carbondale, IL: Southern Illinois University Press.

Smith, A. R. (2007). *The social world of Alcoholics Anonymous: How it works.* New York, NY: iUniverse.

Tonigan, S., Bogenschutz, M. P., & Miller, W. R. (2006). Is alcoholism typology a predictor of both Alcoholics Anonymous affiliation and disaffiliation after treatment? *Journal of Substance Abuse Treatment, 30*(4), 323–330.

Trice, H. M. (1957). A study of the process of affiliation with Alcoholics Anonymous. *Quarterly Journal of Studies on Alcohol, 18*, 39–54.

Trice, H. M. (1959). The affiliation motive and readiness to join Alcoholics Anonymous. *Quarterly Journal of Studies on Alcohol, 20*(2), 313–321.

Vaillant, G. (2003). A 60-year follow-up of alcoholic men. *Addiction, 98*(8), 1043–1051.

Wituk, S. A., Shepherd, M. D., Warren, M., & Meissen, G. (2002). Factors contributing to the survival of self-help groups. *American Journal of Community Psychology, 30*(3), 349–366.

You didn't cause it, you can't cure it, and
you can't control it.

AL-ANON SLOGAN

You can't control your feelings and sensations; you
can control your thoughts, impulses, and muscles.

RECOVERY INTERNATIONAL SLOGAN

10

FOUR MODELS OF SELF-HELP RECOVERY GROUPS

THIS CHAPTER DISCUSSES four different types of recovery groups: a twelve-step fellowship, Al-Anon Family Groups; a non-twelve-step, independent group, Recovery International; a group that receives support from affiliation with a larger foundation, Schizophrenics Anonymous; and a twelve-step group that has modified the steps and traditions, Dual Recovery Anonymous. The chapter covers the history, basic program and ideology, relevant research, how meetings are structured for each group, and how to start a new group. All of these groups offer membership without charge; participants may make a donation at meetings, but this is not required.

AL-ANON FAMILY GROUPS

Lois Wilson threw a shoe at her husband and shouted, "Damn your old meetings!" (Al-Anon, 1979). This is the famous scene in which Lois realizes she needs help for herself, and the seeds of Al-Anon begin to sprout. She recognized that all through the years of Bill Wilson's drinking, she had dreamed of being the one to save him. Now, he had been saved, not by her but by the Oxford Groups and what later became the fellowship of Alcoholics Anonymous.

History

The wives of married AA members usually accompanied their husbands to meetings in the first fourteen years of AA's existence; they participated with their husbands in many of the fellowship activities and believed themselves to be in recovery along with the alcoholics (Al-Anon, 1986). Initially, the family groups were part of AA. They had sprung up all over the country wherever AA met and were sometimes referred to as AA Auxiliaries. AA's cofounders realized the need for a separate fellowship for family members; Bill Wilson urged his wife to undertake the formation of the family groups. Lois Wilson and a good friend, Anne B., formed the first group of Al-Anon in Westchester County, New York, in 1949 (Al-Anon, 1986). At first, extending the fellowship across the country meant converting the existing auxiliaries to Al-Anon groups. In 1951, the first World Service Office opened in New York, with eighty-seven groups in the United States, Canada, Australia, South Africa, and Ireland. In 1996, the World Service Office moved to Virginia Beach, Virginia, with a staff of fifty-six. In 2001, Al-Anon celebrated its fiftieth anniversary. Today there are 26,500 registered groups in 130 countries; Al-Anon literature is published in more than thirty different languages. Al-Anon World Service publishes an extensive library of books, brochures, and media, available from its online store. Its daily meditation book, *One Day at a Time in Al-Anon* (*ODAT*) has sold more than 5 million copies (http://www.al-anon.org/al-anon-history).

Al-Anon surveys a sample of its 600,000 members every three years. Questions on the most recent survey, in 2012, included demographics, level of involvement, reasons for joining, physical and mental health profile, professionals' involvement, spiritual inclination, and impact (http://www.al-anon.alateen.org/membership-survey). Members who responded (n = 3,232) had an average age of fifty-six, and 91 percent were white, 86 percent were female, 31 percent were college graduates, and 58 percent were married. Forty-four percent were unemployed. Almost all of those who responded attended at least one meeting a week, and the average number of years of continuous membership was 11.9. Ten percent of respondents attended meetings online. The greatest percentage of respondents (36 percent) attended because of a husband's alcoholism. Al-Anon's impact on members was significant along many lines: mental and physical health improved; spiritual life improved; physical, emotional, sexual, and verbal abuse decreased; daily functioning improved; and feelings for the alcoholic changed from "frustrated, anxious, and disappointed" to "loving, excited, and proud." Almost all of the respondents had been referred to Al-Anon by a professional helper, 80 percent by a counselor or therapist.

Program

Al-Anon Family Groups was the first organization of many to adapt AA's Twelve Steps and Twelve Traditions for its membership (see box 10.1). A comparison of these steps with those of AA will show that they are relatively the same except for the word "others" in the last step. The same kinds of minimal changes can be found in the twelve steps of other "Anonymous" groups, such as Narcotics Anonymous, Overeaters Anonymous, and Cocaine Anonymous. For example, for NA, the first

BOX 10.1
AL-ANON TWELVE STEPS

1. We admitted we were powerless over alcohol—that our lives had become unmanageable.
2. Came to believe that a Power greater than ourselves could restore us to sanity.
3. Made a decision to turn our will and our lives over to the care of God as we understood Him.
4. Made a searching and fearless moral inventory of ourselves.
5. Admitted to God, to ourselves, and to another human being the exact nature of our wrongs.
6. Were entirely ready to have God remove all these defects of character.
7. Humbly asked Him to remove our shortcomings.
8. Made a list of all persons we had harmed, and became willing to make amends to them all.
9. Made direct amends to such people wherever possible, except when to do so would injure them or others.
10. Continued to take personal inventory and when we were wrong promptly admitted it.
11. Sought through prayer and meditation to improve our conscious contact with God as we understood Him, praying only for knowledge of His will for us and the power to carry that out.
12. Having had a spiritual awakening as the result of these steps, we tried to carry this message to others, and to practice these principles in all our affairs.

Al-Anon (1981, p. 3).

step says "over our addiction" rather than "over alcohol," and the last step says to "carry this message to addicts."

For the same Anonymous groups, traditions have also been used virtually unchanged. This is true for Al-Anon (see box 10.2).

Involvement in Al-Anon on the part of a family member of an active alcoholic can improve the lives of both (McBride, 1992; Wright & Scott, 1978). When Al-Anon members applies the program to themselves, they are able to detach from the alcoholic and allow the drinking person to experience the consequences of his or her illness, thus becoming more able to recognize the alcoholic's need for help from treatment or a recovery group. But more than this, the spouse who can detach from the effects of the illness can also free energy to remain supportive of the alcoholic, especially if he or she is making an effort at sobriety. Research indicates that family

BOX 10.2
AL-ANON TWELVE TRADITIONS

1. Our common welfare should come first; personal progress for the greatest number depends upon unity.
2. For our group purpose there is but one authority—a loving God as He may express Himself in our group conscience. Our leaders are but trusted servants—they do not govern.
3. The relatives of alcoholics, when gathered together for mutual aid, may call themselves an Al-Anon Family Group, provided that, as a group, they have no other affiliation. The only requirement for membership is that there be a problem of alcoholism in a relative or friend.
4. Each group should be autonomous, except in matters affecting another group or Al-Anon or AA as a whole.
5. Each Al-Anon Family Group has but one purpose: to help families of alcoholics. We do this by practicing the Twelve Steps of AA ourselves, by encouraging and understanding our alcoholic relatives, and by welcoming and giving comfort to families of alcoholics.
6. Our Family Groups ought never endorse, finance or lend our name to any outside enterprise, lest problems of money, property and prestige divert us from our primary spiritual aim. Although a separate entity, we should always co-operate with Alcoholics Anonymous.
7. Every group ought to be fully self-supporting, declining outside contributions.
8. Al-Anon Twelfth Step work should remain forever non-professional, but our service centers may employ special workers.
9. Our groups, as such, ought never be organized; but we may create service boards or committees directly responsible to those they serve.
10. The Al-Anon Family Groups have no opinion on outside issues; hence our name ought never be drawn into public controversy.
11. Our public relations policy is based on attraction rather than promotion; we need always maintain personal anonymity at the level of press, radio, films, and TV. We need guard with special care the anonymity of all AA members.
12. Anonymity is the spiritual foundation of all our Traditions, ever reminding us to place principles above personalities.

Al-Anon (1981, pp. 83–84).

support contributes to successful treatment of the alcoholic, but the support offered by the group is mainly for the Al-Anon member (McBride, 1992). One of the first things the new Al-Anon member learns is that he or she is not responsible for the drinking. For some reason, family members often feel that there is something they have done to cause it and that there is something they should to do to stop it. The drinking party may be telling them they are at fault. "If you would stop criticizing me all the time, I wouldn't be getting drunk," the drinker may say. It is true that criticizing the alcoholic makes things worse, as the alcoholic is unable to change on his or her own. New knowledge of how the brain works explains that the alcoholic is unable to overcome the addiction without assistance, and no amount of admonishment by a family member will change that.

The habit of trying to control the alcoholic has become almost second nature to his or her family. One of many Al-Anon jokes is: "If an alcoholic says something in the forest and there's no Al-Anon there to hear him, is he still wrong?" (http://www.soberrecovery.com/forums/recovery-follies/12686-alanon-jokes.html). Jokes like this treat humorously some of the themes family members have to work on repeatedly in their recovery. No one understands this more than fellow Al-Anon members. The typical Al-Anon member is a spouse and is female; statistics from the Al-Anon survey mentioned above reveal that 47 percent of Al-Anon alcoholic partners are in AA, and another 41 percent are still drinking.

That the *ODAT* has sold 5 million copies would not surprise any Al-Anon member. This daily meditation book is used in meetings and sits beside the reading chair or bed of almost every member. Each day's meditation covers one page and contains a spiritual quotation. In the back of the book, there is an index of subjects and the meditations for each. For example, the first subject is "acceptance," with seven numbers leading to pages on that subject. The first reading on this subject is about "accepting the fact that we have no authority or power over any other human being. If we accept this as truth, "we would not try to compel the drinker to do what we want him to (Al-Anon, 1982, p. 32).

In my earlier book (Kurtz, 1997), I discussed how various twelve-step fellowships define the problem. AA, for example, defines the alcoholic's problem, in part, as addiction to alcohol. Alcohol use gradually takes over alcoholics' lives, and in trying to regain control, they lose it completely until they finally have to admit powerlessness, surrender, and ask for help from a power greater than the self. Some people see the concept of powerlessness as requiring that members admit to being powerless over everything, but this misses the point. The first step requires that alcoholics admit powerlessness over alcohol, a power they have already lost. AA goes further in problem definition: "Selfishness—self-centeredness! That, we think, is the root of our troubles" (AA, 1939/1976, p. 62). The goal is to "quit playing God" (p. 63) and decide to "turn our lives and our will over to the care of God, as we understood Him" (p. 59).

For families of alcoholics, the problem is the breakdown of family life and loss of normal role behavior by the drinking partners or parents, which leads to changes in roles of other members. Eventually, the family regains equilibrium by denying the problem or by isolating the drinking person and taking over his or her previous role in the family. Despite the new sense of equilibrium, the stresses brought on by the alcoholic's actions often become an obsession. Al-Anon addresses all of this by teaching family members, first, that they are powerless over the alcoholic and, second, that they must detach from the obsession to control and instead create a spiritual way of life for themselves (Al-Anon, 1981; Al-Anon, 1965/1986). The effect of one member's alcoholism on the rest of the family is illustrated in Lin's story (box 10.3).

In 1957, Al-Anon World Service formed Alateen for twelve-to-nineteen-year-old children of alcoholics (Al-Anon, 1986). The World Service Office assigned staff to help with the formation of groups and literature, and by 1960, there were one hundred groups around the country. Today there are more than one thousand Alateen meetings in the world. Alateen members keep the focus on themselves and discuss

BOX 10.3
LIN'S STORY

I was born in 1941 to a wonderful family. My mother was a brilliant Oberlin College-educated woman who knew the world of music and nature. I idolized my dad and loved being with him even though he was a heavy drinker. I was his watch dog and spent time at the "Joint," lounge where he and his political buddies hung out. As time went on, my father's drinking got worse. One evening, Dad was carried into the house before Christmas by four men who carried him up to his bedroom on the second floor of the house. He was passed out; I thought he was dead. That is when I asked my mother about Dad's drinking being a problem, and her response was he was just a heavy social drinker, and he hadn't eaten anything, so the alcohol affected him more than it would otherwise. At school, I was in a class called Effective Living. It touched on areas like alcoholism and birth control. A man came and talked about his alcoholism; he told my dad's story. I left the class in tears.

When I went to college, I was very shy, and I had to force myself to talk. At first, I made a point not to drink or smoke. Well, there was this cool place on campus across from the old gym called Ted's. Ted's had high-back wooden booths, and you could see the smoke rise as you walked in the door. Well, you guessed it—I learned to smoke. Shortly thereafter, I was invited to frat parties and "TGIFs." I was shy and decided to try a beer. I didn't like the taste, but I found out I didn't feel so anxious anymore. I never drank daily, but when I did drink, it was often too much.

My drinking continued but only at school. Between my junior and senior year, I got married to the captain of the football team. We were both shy, and both of us drank at parties. Just after our first son was born, my father ended up in the hospital with

(*Continued*)

the worst case of DTs I have ever seen. We took twelve-hour shifts with him in a classroom, as he was so loud they couldn't keep him in a regular hospital room. I remember walking into the room, and he said, "You are over twenty-one, go get me a bottle." He knew that was the only way the shakes would stop. His liver was so bad they didn't medicate him. He was in and out of a coma over the next month. Following that, he was in and out of the state hospital for the next two years. My mother moved in with us because they lost their house.

I was first introduced to Al-Anon at this time at Christ Church. I was amazed to find out that it wasn't about fixing my dad but about changing me. It also showed me that I wasn't the only one who had to deal with someone they loved having the disease of alcoholism. At that time, most of us were very afraid to say any family member was alcoholic. The stigma in the late '50s through the '70s was much greater than it is now. Al-Anon gave me a safe place to go and not feel shame. It also taught me I was not responsible for Dad's drinking.

I knew at this time I didn't want to end up like my dad. He had the form of brain damage from alcohol where he couldn't learn and retain what he had learned. Man, I didn't want to go there, but I still drank to excess. My last drinking episode was at a teacher party. All week, I had waited to go drinking. I planned to have a babysitter, and I was going to get drunk and happy. I remember sitting by the door of the house where the party was. One drink, another, another, and another, and I wasn't getting happy no matter how much I drank. Instead, I became suicidal. I came home and at two in the morning was sitting on my neighbor's fence looking for a gravel truck to jump in front of.

Thirty-two years ago, I moved away. My marriage ended after twenty years. I knew one person well and knew I needed support. I remembered that AA said the only requirement for membership was "a desire to stop drinking." I did want to stop. Everyone said, "You are just like your dad." I didn't want to die at age fifty-six from alcoholism and cause all kinds of trauma to people who loved me. I decided the fastest way to meet people was AA and group therapy. I did both. I needed all the support I could get. My story is not the ordinary road to sobriety. Thank God, I was given the insight to learn from others so that I didn't have to reach a horrible bottom.

Another big turnaround came two years after I moved, when one of my new AA friends said, "I have to talk to you, and it may cost us our friendship, but I can't lie to you. I am in love with you." She bent down and kissed my cheek. My mind and body went places it had never been. She had a more severe drinking problem than I. I told her if she relapsed and didn't get help, I would leave, that I wouldn't live through it again. She didn't drink after that. We attended meetings together for twenty-eight years until her death three years ago.

I love that the AA and Al-Anon focus is on me changing and me not thinking I can change everybody else. I like having friends who are funny, intelligent, sensitive, and open. Twelve-step programs are a great place to find those folks how they can apply the twelve steps to cope with living with an alcoholic parent. Like their adult Al-Anon parent, they learn to detach from the drinker's problems while continuing to love the person. All Alateen groups are sponsored by an adult Al-Anon member who attends every meeting.

Research

Al-Anon has not been studied extensively, but existing research indicates that Al-Anon membership by families leads to better outcomes for the alcoholics in treatment and that Al-Anon participation contributes to improved mental health in its members. In one study (Timko, Young, & Moos, 2012), remission rates for alcoholics in treatment whose family members attended Al-Anon, were nearly double those of the patients whose families did not participate. After reviewing the literature on Al-Anon, the researchers recommend that practitioners work harder to involve families in the group earlier in patients' treatment and that professionals help Al-Anon recruit more minority members (Al-Anon's current membership is 91 percent white). Professional efforts along these lines would likely be very effective, because Al-Anon's survey indicates that almost all of its members were referred to the group by a professional.

Meeting Structure

Al-Anon suggests the following meeting structure. A chairman opens the meeting with a welcome message followed by the Serenity Prayer, an introduction of a topic for discussion, and encouragement for those present to take part in the discussion. The meeting closes with the Serenity Prayer or some other prayer (Al-Anon, 1966/1984). Al-Anon groups sometimes schedule open meetings for interested parties who do not qualify as members. Usually, the program for an open meeting centers on a talk by a visiting member or professional.

Starting a Group

"The relatives and friends of alcoholics, when gathered together for mutual aid, may call themselves an Al-Anon Family Group, provided that, as a group, they have no other affiliation. The only requirement for membership is that there be a problem of alcoholism in a relative or friend" (http://www.al-anon.org). Eligible members may begin a new group by deciding on a meeting place and contacting the World Service Office to register it. Once the group is registered, Al-Anon will send a starter kit with brochures and newsletters. The new group must contact the local district to have itself listed in the meeting guide for the local area.

RECOVERY INTERNATIONAL

Recovery International started out in the early 1930s as an aftercare group for the patients treated by psychiatrist Abraham A. Low at Illinois State Psychiatric Institute. Low taught his patients his original terminology for discussing symptoms that he believed led to relapse, holding that a new language could change both thinking and behavior. Unlike most psychiatrists of the day, he saw some of his patients in groups.

History

In 1937, Low encouraged his patients to incorporate as a public educational society called Recovery, Inc. (Low, 1943/1991). Thirty former patients of the Illinois State Psychiatric Institute attended the first meeting, on November 7, 1937. It met monthly thereafter and focused specifically on changing the state commitment law, which required that persons admitted to the state hospital be arrested and taken to the hospital as though they were criminals. Recovery, Inc., members and Low thought that being arrested and taken to the hospital contributed to stigma.

The group pressured the Illinois Psychiatric Society to study the need for changing the law, spread its organizational base to the state hospitals, and gave public lectures and radio talks. This went on for four years while a bill changing the state's commitment law passed both houses of the state legislature and went before the governor. During this same time, members worked on reducing the stigma of mental illness in other ways, mainly by speaking to audiences. All along, members continued to practice the recovery techniques taught by Low for their own mental health. Ultimately, the governor of Illinois vetoed the new commitment bill. Low, meanwhile, had been pressured by his fellow psychiatrists to abandon the group practice he had begun. Feeling that his experiment in establishing the group was successful, he expected to be able to spread this idea to others at state mental hospitals. But his attempt to initiate Recovery groups inside hospitals failed. When he realized this, Low, in despair, "liquidated" his group in 1941. The members refused to give up, however, and continued to meet as a "self-help" collective. Low had not intended to invent a self-help association, but he did, and it was to be one of the longest-lasting and most original developments of the twentieth century. Low gave the organization his blessing, kept in touch, and wrote three or four books on his techniques for the self-help groups to use (Low, 1950).

Program

Recovery International, as the group has been known since 2007, defines members' problems as episodes of either fearful or angry temper, which, if left unattended, could precipitate another breakdown and hospitalization. (Recovery rarely speaks in terms of diagnoses, nor does it use usual psychological terminology.) In his aftercare meetings with patients at the Illinois State Psychiatric Institute, Low taught them to use his own set of terms as a means of changing thoughts and behaviors, which he called "will training." Will training is an early example of cognitive-behavioral methods in which members change the way they think and behave by spotting episodes of temper. Members combat fearful temper and low feelings by "moving the muscles" and "doing the thing that you fear to do" (Low, 1950). Angry temper is alleviated by reinterpreting situations. For example, another person is doing something you do not like. You can spot this as angry temper and tell yourself that the situation is trivial, not worth having a spell of temper over.

Today Recovery International lists six hundred community-based meetings in the United States and seven other countries. It also sponsors fifteen online meetings. The organization supporting it is Abraham Low Self-Help Systems (http://www.lowselfhelpsystems.org/about/history.asp). Recovery International's website features a link to online ordering for books and other resources, such as power tool cards for learning Low's method, numerous books by Low including his *Mental Health Through Will Training*, compact discs containing his lectures, and a new book, *RI Discovery: Participant Workbook*. The power tool cards and workbook are valuable for learning Low's terminology, which members need in order to give panel examples in meetings and, even more, to use in their own lives.

The question of how Recovery International and twelve-step groups work for people who want to attend both is a good one. Are they compatible or incompatible? Cliff Brown, who has attended Recovery, Emotions Anonymous, and Emotional Health Anonymous groups, discusses this subject on the Recovery International website (http://www.lowselfhelpsystems.org/system/our-method-vs-12-step-programs.asp);

> Recovery International and 12-step programs have much in common from a structural point of view. Both are international in scope and essentially free. A basket is passed during meetings, where one is invited to make a donation, but no fee is required to attend. Meetings generally last from one and one-half to two hours. In addition, both programs utilize reading from program texts and encourage the use of helpful sayings and slogans in one's daily life. Also, both stress, perhaps in different ways, the importance of changing one's thinking and attitude and recognize the value of self-awareness and self-examination.
>
> Another important commonality is that both offer the participant encouragement, support and acceptance as they struggle to overcome their difficulties. Finally, Recovery International and the 12-step program urge the attendee to read and study various books and literature between meetings and point out the necessity of practicing program principles in one's daily life if one wants to get well.

Differences between the two also exist. One significant difference is in meeting structure. Although both types of groups have structure, twelve-step groups can have a variety of structures, such as open talks, twelve-step study, open and closed discussion, topical discussions, and others. Recovery International meetings, on the other hand, are all structured the same way and much more precisely: introduction, reading, panel examples, followed by analysis of the examples. In addition, Brown writes:

> The 12-step program is rooted, to a marked degree, in the belief that by surrendering or turning over one's will, symptoms or problems to a power greater than oneself (or God if one chooses) inner progress in the form of reduced difficulties, serenity, contentment and peace of mind are obtained. Recovery International, through what is known as the Recovery system, on the other hand, emphasizes more of a "down-to-earth" cognitive-behavioral approach for dealing with one's problems, stressing the importance of using one's will, in a positive manner, to help oneself. Recovery International, however, does recognize the limitations of the will in that we cannot control the "outer environment."

Although Low thought that introducing religion and spiritual principles was not helpful for his process to work, Brown points out that Recovery International's focus on using the will to overcome troubles also instructs members to strive for averageness, to think of the group rather than oneself, and to achieve humility. Twelve-step programs aim for the same kind of outcome in their instruction to adopt a "willingness" to work the program of recovery. Thus, both approaches teach that one must use willpower appropriately and that participants need to reduce self-centeredness.

Research

Recovery International has been the subject of much research. The most recent is an evaluation by Susan Pickett and her colleagues at the Department of Psychiatry, University of Illinois at Chicago (Pickett, Phillips, & Kraus, 2011). This three-year study followed new members over time to assess satisfaction and knowledge of how to use the method. Satisfaction levels were high, with respondents liking the positive environment of meetings and the skills of peer leaders. The researchers tested knowledge of the Recovery method using a seventeen-item multiple-choice questionnaire. The average score was 13 out of a possible 17. Researchers tested members' ability to use the method by asking them to give a four-part example in each interview. On average, most respondents were able to give three out of four parts of an example.

Meeting Structure

Recovery International meetings follow a pattern as follows: reading Low's book, panel examples from a selection of members, then discussion among members present. Contributions and examples follow the same plan: describe an instance in which an ordinary event led you to be "worked up," explaining what happened and what triggered temper and symptoms; report the symptoms you experienced, both physical and mental; report your spotting of fearful or angry temper and the Recovery tools you used to help yourself; begin with "Before I had my Recovery training..." and describe the temperamental response and symptoms you would have experienced in former days, what would have happened then versus what happened now (Abraham Low Self-Help Systems, 2009).

An example that I reported on in a Recovery meeting years ago illustrates. We were having our house painted. It was summer, and the gardens were in bloom, which is important to me. I looked out the window and observed two of the painters washing their brushes and emptying paint cans in the back of the yard in one of the flower gardens. Right away, I began to work myself up into angry temper. How dare they pour their toxic paint into my flower garden! I wish I could say that I spotted my temperamental response in time to subdue it, but I didn't. I charged out to the garden and gave them a piece of my mind. Later, I spotted that I had worked myself up into an angry temper. I reminded myself of several Recovery tools: first, recognizing that this was an ordinary situation that was "distressing but not dangerous"; seeing further that "my feelings should be expressed and my temper suppressed"; realizing that "there is no right or wrong in the trivialities of everyday life"; and ultimately, understanding that "people do things that annoy us, not to annoy us." Before I learned Recovery practice, I would have gone back into the house, called the painting contractor, and complained about his men. Instead, I spotted my temperamental response and let it go. If I had spotted it sooner, I would have behaved "like a cultured person" and calmly asked the painters to wash the brushes somewhere else.

After the panel presentation, meeting participants go around the room and comment on the story. In doing so, they also use Recovery tools. The various quotes in my example above and others would come from members as the conversation continued. In my experience, members must comment using the Recovery terminology, and in this way, it becomes more familiar to them. Using Low's vocabulary requires practice and reading his book. Group leaders have preparation by the organization in leading groups and using the will-training process.

Starting a Group

Although professionals are welcome to assist with the development of Recovery International groups, only volunteers who have been *patients* are allowed to lead groups. Anyone interested in forming new communities should contact the Recovery International home office in Chicago to learn how to do this (http://www.lowselfhelpsystems.org/system/our-method.asp).

SCHIZOPHRENICS ANONYMOUS

In 1970, Joanne Verbanic opened the door of a moving car and started to jump out because voices were telling her to kill herself. Fifteen years later, she founded Schizophrenics Anonymous (SA) in Detroit. In between those dates, she had stable periods working for Ford Motor Credit, interspersed with periods of psychosis for which she had to enter a psychiatric hospital. The last psychotic episode happened in 1984. She founded SA in 1985. At that time, there were no groups solely for people with the most serious psychiatric diagnosis possible; the need was great.

History

SA began with Verbanic's offer to do volunteer work for the Mental Health Association in Michigan (MHAM) (Salem, Reischl, & Randall, 2008). She did not intend to start a group, but after her meetings with MHAM leaders, she put an ad in a suburban paper seeking other people with schizophrenia. Two people showed up, and they began meeting in public places—a park, a local restaurant. Later, when the group grew larger, the association offered meeting space. MHAM also assisted with a pamphlet that informed possible members about SA, which Verbanic mailed to all the psychiatrists in Detroit. Attendance grew as she made public appearances talking about her diagnosis. By the end of the fifth year, members of the first group had begun eight more groups in southeastern Michigan. Verbanic's fearless honesty about having what is probably the most stigmatized medical diagnosis possible was key to her success in recruiting members and starting new groups.

At the end of SA's sixth year, Verbanic was overwhelmed by the demands of the growing organization and asked MHAM for help with staffing, funding, and materials. MHAM obtained grant money for this, and the SA group moved from internal leadership development to a shared model in which the association hired staff to help begin new groups (see chapter 5). By the end of the twelfth year, 40 percent of SA's groups had professional leadership. The budding association continued to experience rapid growth, needing more formal organizational control by the professionals involved in leadership. As of 2013, SA had 150 groups meeting in thirty-one states, with additional groups in Australia, Brazil, Canada, Mexico, France, India, and Venezuela.

In January 2008, a steering committee of consumers, families, and providers across the United States created a national organization dedicated to improving the lives of people with schizophrenia and related disorders. In February, the committee named the new organization Schizophrenia and Related Disorders Alliance of America (SARDAA). In March, it formed a board of directors and hired a part-time consultant to build the organization. In May 2008 SARDAA was incorporated as a nonstock corporation in Maryland. SARDAA's mission is to promote hope and recovery for people with schizophrenia and related disorders, to raise awareness and decrease stigma surrounding the illness, and to ensure that services are available to those in need. One of its programs is to provide technical support to SA. The organization maintains a website with links to SA, literature sales and publishing, a blog, a weekly newsletter, and other resources, including SA's "Blue Book" (SARDAA, 2010).

Program

SA is an example of an international self-help recovery association that is supported by a national organization with professional leadership and fundraising capacity. SA's name may seem to imply that it is a twelve-step fellowship, but it is not. SA defines itself as a "self-help peer support group for persons who have schizophrenia or a schizophrenia-related illness." Related illnesses include illnesses that "have psychotic symptoms, including hallucinations and delusions, such as schizoaffective disorder, bipolar disorder, psychotic depression, and psychosis" (SARDAA, 2010, p. 3). The founders modeled the program after AA but reduced the steps to six and rewrote them (see boxes 10.4 and 10.5).

The SA understanding of schizophrenia involves both the medical and the recovery models. It views schizophrenia as: a brain-based biological, genetic, and structural disorder that impairs psychological, cognitive, social, and emotional functioning" (SARDAA, 2010, p. 2). However, it also holds that recovery is possible and that all people can engage in recovery regardless of symptom severity or other circumstances. Members define recovery as living up to one's potential and finding a place for oneself in the world. As Randall and Salem (2007) point out, SA gives people with the illness something no other group can give: role models, people recovering from schizophrenia. It is the one place where people with the diagnosis tell their stories of recovery. These are told in regular meetings, in the Blue Book, in newsletters, in public forums, and on the SA website. Before SA, people with schizophrenia were typically depicted as hopeless and incurable, with little or no

BOX 10.4
SCHIZOPHRENICS ANONYMOUS SIX STEPS

1. I surrender...I admit I need help. I can't do it alone.
2. I choose...I choose to be well. I take full responsibility for my choices and realize the choices I make directly influence the quality of my days.
3. I believe...I now come to believe that I have been provided with great inner resources and I will use these resources to help myself and others.
4. I forgive...I forgive myself for all the mistakes I have made. I also forgive and release everyone who has injured or harmed me in any way.
5. I understand...I now understand that erroneous, self-defeating thinking contributes to my problems, failures, unhappiness and fears. I am ready to have my belief system altered so my life can be transformed.
6. I decide...I make a decision to turn my life over to the care of a higher power/God, AS I UNDERSTAND that higher power/God, surrendering my will and false beliefs. I ask to be changed in depth.

SARDAA (2010, p. 5).

access to alternative descriptions. Stigma motivated anyone who could do so to hide the illness; those passing for normal were not going to tell their stories to the world.

Research

Randall and Salem (2007) identify two other advantages provided by SA. One is the availability of opportunities to participate in meaningful social roles, such as group leader, newsletter writer, meeting participant, organizer of conferences, and one-on-one helper of new members. Second, members have a place to go for social support, connection to others, and a sense of belonging. Like other recovery groups and social agencies using the recovery philosophy, SA provides hope to people who have not had hope in their lives and does so precisely for people with the most serious form of mental health condition.

Meeting Structure

SA meetings begin with reading the SA Statement of Purpose and a selection from the book of affirmations, followed by introductions. The rest of the meeting involves discussion of methods for coping with everyday problems, strategies for handling psychotic symptoms, and discussion of one of the steps. All members have a

BOX 10.5
SCHIZOPHRENICS ANONYMOUS GUIDING PRINCIPLES

1. The only requirement for SA membership is the desire to recover from a schizophrenia related illness.
2. There are no dues for SA membership, although donations may be accepted to cover SA group expenses or special events.
3. Everything said at SA meetings is confidential.
4. SA members should remain anonymous, except those who wish to work on special issues; SA members and leaders should place principles before personalities in all matters relating to our program.
5. Each group may establish its own meeting format, subject to approval by central SA leadership.
6. Decisions affecting SA as a whole are derived from the group consciousness of its own members; we rely on our Higher Power to work through this process.

SARDAA (2010, p. 7)

chance to talk, and crosstalk is encouraged. The group's leader encourages participation. Member contributions to the discussion can be about how the SA program has helped them or a problem with which they want help. Meetings end with the Serenity Prayer. SA's Blue Book (SARDAA, 2010) provides an extensive explanation of steps and suggestions for meeting discussions; it also includes variations on meeting formats and topics.

Starting a Group

Individuals who want to start a new SA group can purchase an start-up kit from SARDAA's online store for $250. The kit contains an instruction DVD, electronic copies of all materials, ten Blue Books, a group leader's manual, ten brochures, toll-free participation in quarterly conference calls, and support from a veteran SA leader. The Blue Book gives the following guidelines on starting an SA group:

1. Contact the central office.
2. A skilled veteran guides the caller through the group start-up process.
3. Technical support identifies a local cosponsor, gives aid in finding a meeting place, and offers suggestions for publicizing the group.
4. The central office will refer inquiries from individuals to the new group.

DUAL RECOVERY ANONYMOUS

The fourth type of group to be discussed in this chapter is a twelve-step program that addresses both an addiction and a mental health condition. Dual diagnosis refers to a medical judgment that the individual has both problems. Thirty-seven percent of alcohol abusers and 53 percent of drug abusers also have at least one serious mental illness. Of all people diagnosed as mentally ill, 29 percent abuse either alcohol or drugs (http://www.nmha.org/go/information/get-info/co-occurring-disorders/dual-diagnosis). Many individual, unaffiliated dual diagnosis groups meet at mental health centers and other places convenient to members (Kurtz et al., 1995). One of the largest networks, however, is Dual Recovery Anonymous (DRA).

History

DRA began in Prairie Village, Kansas, in 1989. Its goals were to develop a self-help program based on (1) the principles of the twelve steps, (2) personal experience of dual recovery, and (3) principles of personal freedom and choice. The fellowship has two requirements for membership: "a desire to stop using alcohol or other intoxicating drugs; and a desire to manage emotional or psychiatric illness in a healthy and constructive way" (http://draonline.org).

In the twenty-four years since its founding in 1989, DRA established 880 in-person meetings in all fifty states and five foreign countries: Australia, Canada, Iceland, India, and New Zealand. It uses a modified version of AA's Twelve Steps and Twelve Traditions (see boxes 10.6 and 10.7).

Meeting Structure

DRA meetings follow a format similar to that in other twelve-step fellowships. The typical meeting begins with an opening welcome statement, followed by the Serenity Prayer. Next comes the "preamble" spelling out the purpose of DRA, the requirements for membership, and the type of organization it is, that is, a nonprofessional self-help program with clear boundaries separating it from professionals and their organizations. This is followed by announcements, introductions, and a reading on "accepting differences." Someone then reads "Getting Started in Dual Recovery." The next item is a roundtable discussion in which everyone has a chance to share on the subject of his or her recovery practice. The meeting ends with passing the basket and another recital of the Serenity Prayer.

Starting a Group

To get assistance with beginning a new group of DRA, contact the central office, and go to the website (http://draonline.org) to order a meeting start-up packet. The

BOX 10.6
DUAL RECOVERY ANONYMOUS TWELVE STEPS

1. We admitted we were powerless over our dual illness of chemical dependency and emotional or psychiatric illness—that our lives had become unmanageable.
2. Came to believe that a Higher Power of our understanding could restore us to sanity.
3. Made a decision to turn our will and our lives over to the care of our Higher Power, to help us to rebuild our lives in a positive and caring way.
4. Made a searching and fearless personal inventory of ourselves.
5. Admitted to our Higher Power, to ourselves, and to another human being the exact nature of our liabilities and our assets.
6. Were entirely ready to have our Higher Power remove all our liabilities.
7. Humbly asked our Higher Power to remove these liabilities and to help us to strengthen our assets for recovery.
8. Made a list of all persons we had harmed and became willing to make amends to them all.
9. Made direct amends to such people wherever possible, except when to do so would injure them or others.
10. Continued to take personal inventory and when wrong promptly admitted it, while continuing to recognize our progress in dual recovery.
11. Sought through prayer and meditation to improve our conscious contact with our Higher Power, praying only for knowledge of our Higher Power's will for us and the power to carry that out.
12. Having had a spiritual awakening as a result of these Steps, we tried to carry this message to others who experience dual disorders and to practice these principles in all our affairs.

http://draonline.org/files/steps.pdf

website also offers a directory of meetings, personal stories of members, readings about the fellowship, and questions and answers about combined mental illness and alcohol and drug use.

CONCLUSION

This chapter has summarized what I think are the most salient characteristics in the history and development of four self-help associations. Two of them are among the oldest fellowships: Al-Anon Family Groups and Recovery International. The

BOX 10.7
DUAL RECOVERY ANONYMOUS TWELVE TRADITIONS

1. The primary purpose of DRA is to carry the message of recovery to men and women who experience a dual disorder.
2. DRA has two requirements for membership: a desire to stop using alcohol and other intoxicating drugs, and a desire to manage our emotional or psychiatric illness in a healthy and constructive way.
3. We welcome men and women of all personal beliefs; our program is one of personal freedom and choice.
4. Our groups and service work are guided by the principles of the 12 Steps of DRA.
5. Each group is independent, to better meet the recovery needs of our members. We are sensitive to the well-being and unity of other groups and to DRA as a whole.
6. To maintain our primary purpose, we avoid all outside distractions. We need not become involved in financial entanglements, lend the DRA name for outside activities and issues, or become drawn into public controversy.
7. Every DRA group ought to be self-supporting.
8. DRA is a volunteer, self-help organization. To carry out our service work, we may employ special workers, form committees and coordinate projects.
9. Our individual dual recovery depends on DRA unity. We carry the message through our personal recovery and our service work.
10. DRA is a non-professional program. We do not provide chemical dependency, mental health or other social services. DRA has no opinion regarding the appropriate use of medications or other methods of managing our symptoms.
11. In DRA we share an equal partnership in dual recovery. Our traditions and service work help us maintain the integrity of our program, to provide for others and to enhance the unity of DRA as a whole.
12. Personal anonymity is the right of every DRA member. We practice anonymity at the level of public media.

---

http://draonline.org/files/trads.pdf

other two are relatively new groups, just starting out and with the usual growing pains. It's worth mentioning that three have administrative staff and offices. Running an international network of self-help recovery groups is not a task for volunteers. Nevertheless, these associations charge no dues or fees for the services they provide.

The next chapter addresses the subject of advocacy and how twelve-step groups foster advocacy and community service in spite of their traditions. The early history of AA and the development of the National Council on Alcoholism and Drug Dependency demonstrate how AA members have influenced public policy and awareness. Recent efforts to influence policy come from Faces & Voices of Recovery. The chapter also discusses advocacy organizations in the mental health field: the well-known National Alliance on Mental Illness and consumer-run survivor groups such as MindFreedom International.

REFERENCES

AA. (1939/1976). *Alcoholics Anonymous: The story of how many thousands of men and women have recovered from alcoholism*. New York, NY: AA World Services.

Abraham Low Self-Help Systems. (2009). *RI discovery: Participant workbook*. Chicago, IL: Abraham Low Self-Help Systems.

Al-Anon. (1965/1986). *Al-Anon faces alcoholism* (2nd ed.). New York, NY: Al-=Anon Family Groups.

Al-Anon. (1966/1984). *Al-Anon Family Groups* (rev. ed.). New York, NY: Al-Anon Family Groups.

Al-Anon. (1979). *Lois remembers: Memoirs of the co-founder of Al-Anon and the wife of the co-founder of Alcoholics Anonymous*. New York, NY: Al-Anon Family Groups.

Al-Anon. (1981). *Al-Anon's twelve steps and twelve traditions*. New York, NY: Al-Anon Family Groups.

Al-Anon. (1982). *One day at a time in Al-Anon*. New York, NY: Al-Anon Family Groups.

Al-Anon. (1986). *First steps: Al-Anon… 35 years of beginnings*. New York, NY: Al-Anon Family Groups.

Kurtz, L. F. (1997). *Self-help and support groups: A handbook for practitioners*. Thousand Oaks, CA: Sage.

Kurtz, L. F., Garvin, C. D., Hill, E. M., Pollio, D., McPherson, S., & Powell, T. J. (1995). Involvement in Alcoholics Anonymous by persons with dual disorders. *Alcoholism Treatment Quarterly, 12*(4), 1–18.

Low, A. A. (1943/1991). *Mental illness, stigma and self-help*. Glencoe, IL: Willet Publishing.

Low, A. A. (1950). *Mental health through will training*. Glencoe, IL: Willet Publishing.

McBride, J. L. (1992). Assessing the Al-Anon component of Alcoholics Anonymous. *Alcoholism Treatment Quarterly, 8*(4), 57–65.

Pickett, S., Phillips, H., & Kraus, D. (2011). *Recovery International group meeting evaluation: Final report*. Available at http://www.lowselfhelpsystems.org/documents/ri_final_report_3.1.11.pdf

Randall, K. W., & Salem, D. A. (2007). Mutual-help groups and recovery: The influence of settings on the participant's experience of recovery. In R. O. Ralph & P. W. Corrigan (Eds.), *Recovery in mental illness: Broadening our understanding of wellness* (pp. 173–206). Washington, DC: American Psychological Association.

Salem, D. A., Reischl, T. M., & Randall, K. W. (2008). The effect of professional partnership on the development of a mutual-help organization. *American Journal of Community Psychology, 42*, 179–191.

SARDAA. (2010). *Schizophrenics Anonymous self-help peer support group* [Blue Book]. Houston, TX: SARDAA.

Timko, C., Young, L. B., & Moos, R. H. (2012). Al-Anon Family Groups: Origins, conceptual basis, outcomes, and research opportunities. *Journal of Groups in Addiction & Recovery, 7*, 279–296.

Wright, K. E., & Scott, T. B. (1978). The relationship of wives' treatment to the drinking status of alcoholics. *Journal of Studies on Alcohol, 39*(9), 1577–1581.

3

[O]n Market Street where the march crested a bridge revealing recovering people as far as the eyes could see before me and behind me.

WHITE (2010)

11

RECOVERY GROUPS AND ADVOCACY

THIS CHAPTER ACQUAINTS the reader with advocacy among people recovering from addictions and mental health conditions. As noted in chapter 2, the two fields are quite separate when it comes to advocacy, this despite the reality that stigma and the lack of appropriate services afflict both groups in the same way. One of the myths about the addictions field is that people who claim to be powerless over alcohol, the first step in a twelve-step fellowship, are incapable of becoming empowered. Read here about the country's oldest advocacy group in the addictions field, the National Council on Alcoholism and Drug Dependency, to learn how empowered recovering people have been all along and are becoming despite adherence to the first step. I've also included an explanation of the tenth and eleventh AA traditions and how they are misunderstood with regard to member actions in local communities and on a national and growing international level. Following that are descriptions of the National Alliance on Mental Illness and the consumer/survivor advocacy movement among former and current mental health patients.

NATIONAL COUNCIL ON ALCOHOLISM AND DRUG DEPENDENCY

Some people think that the "disease concept of alcoholism" came from AA, but it didn't. It really emerged on a national platform because of Marty Mann, recovering alcoholic, member of AA, and founder of the National Council on Alcoholism (NCA) (and Drug Dependence, NCADD) (Brown & Brown, 2001). She used the disease concept as an organizing metaphor for the growing movement and as a way to divert the public from the idea of "drunkenness solely in terms of sin and moral degeneracy" (White, 1998, p. 198). Mann stopped drinking in 1939, and in 1940, she was one of the first women in AA. Her story, "Women Suffer Too," was the woman's story in the second and third editions of the AA Big Book (AA, 1955; AA, 1976). She was aware of AA's eleventh tradition, which says, "Our public relations policy is based on attraction rather than promotion; we need always maintain personal anonymity at the level of press, radio and film" (AA, 1976, p. 564), but she decided that to be effective, she should violate that tradition and speak publicly as an AA member, including in press releases and spots on movie newsreels, to educate the public. Many AA members speak up like this but, in deference to the eleventh tradition, do not reveal their AA status. In her role as the founder of one of the oldest advocacy organizations in the country, Mann gave more than two hundred speeches each year, telling her own recovery story and explaining the disease concept of alcoholism (Brown & Brown, 2001).

Before Mann and the NCA, the word "alcoholism" was virtually unknown; instead, it was called "inebriety." Inebriety then, as with drug addiction today, was considered a criminal act that needed punishment. Mann would say, "Arrests of persons with this disease are about as effective for cure as arresting a cancer patient for the criminal act of having cancer" (Brown & Brown, 2001, p. 175). She would point out how much less it cost to treat an alcoholic than to put him or her into jail. She would tell her audience that after spending thousands of dollars to keep the alcoholic in a penal institution, he or she would be released just as addicted and sick as he was the day he went in.

Mann joined the staff of the Yale Center of Alcohol Studies and, with its backing, in 1944 formed the National Committee for Education on Alcoholism (NCEA). Her goals were to educate health professionals, to establish information centers in every state, and to promote treatment for alcoholics. AA's just-established traditions forbade political activity by the fellowship, but as AA members spread across the country in the same years as the NCEA, this made it seem as though the two organizations were functioning hand-in-hand, one serving the individual alcoholic, the other informing the public and influencing policy, and both having roughly the same people as members. From NCADD's website comes this introduction:

> For nearly 70 years, NCADD has been a valuable resource for millions of people struggling with addiction. Our founder, Marty Mann, was a true pioneer. Marty got sober in the rooms of Alcoholics Anonymous (AA). When AA was just getting started in 1935, Marty's sponsor was AA Co-founder, Bill Wilson. Marty exuded courage and unwavering belief in the dignity of all people. She worked tirelessly to provide education to raise the awareness of addiction across our society. (http://www.ncadd.org/index.php/about-ncadd/about-ncadd)

The website welcome goes on to say that Mann made two decisions when she started the NCEA. To be a credible agent for change, (1) it would need the involvement of the medical and scientific community, and (2) it must offer professional counseling in order to change attitudes and understanding. When Mann first conceived of the idea for the organization, she came up with "three simple ideas" that still inspire the program today: (1) alcoholism is a disease, (2) the alcoholic can be helped and is worth helping, and (3) alcoholism is a public health problem and therefore a public responsibility. These are true today, except that her organization now includes drug dependency.

Mann remained director of NCEA (later NCA and then NCADD) until 1972. During that time, there were significant accomplishments: by 1953, three thousand hospitals began offering care to alcoholics where almost none did before; in 1956, the American Medical Association urged hospitals to accept alcoholics for treatment; in 1957, a Roper poll showed that 53 percent of the public viewed alcoholism as a disease, compared with 6 percent in 1943; in 1963, the American Public Health Association identified alcoholism as a treatable illness; in 1969, President Johnson signed the Public Services Amendment Act, which awarded funds for staffing community mental health centers to provide specialized facilities for treating alcoholics and other addicts; in 1970, the Comprehensive Alcohol Abuse and Alcoholism Prevention Treatment and Rehabilitation Act (Hughes Act) passed and signed into law; in 1973, US investigators discovered fetal alcohol syndrome, a significant contributor to developmental disabilities affecting intellect and behavior; in 1974, Congress created the National Institute on Drug Abuse (NIDA); in 1976, NCADD conducted Operation Understanding, a news conference in Washington, D.C., where fifty-two prominent individuals publicly acknowledged their recovery from alcoholism; in 1980, NCADD affiliates numbered more than two hundred.

The list of accomplishments goes on. Those mentioned above are a selection of public victories in the alcoholism and, later, drug abuse fields that happened during Mann's lifetime. NCADD will soon celebrate seventy years of public information and advocacy. As far as I know, none of its leadership over the years has announced publicly membership in the AA fellowship, but I would guess that many, if not most, follow in the same footsteps as the founder. NCADD has a pamphlet entitled "Advocacy with Anonymity," encouraging recovering people to engage in advocacy and public service without violating twelve-step traditions.

ADVOCACY, ANONYMITY, THE FIRST STEP, AND THE TWELVE TRADITIONS

There has been an insidious myth about twelve-step fellowships, which is that participants in such groups immerse themselves in closed recovery systems that discourage reinstatement into the wider community and form a barrier to personal and political empowerment (Beauchamp, 1980; Williams, 1992). For example, Beauchamp (1980, p. 68) wrote: "The elaborate and striking emphasis in AA on withdrawal from the community could only make sense to a culture supremely confident that alcohol and alcohol policy are not an issue in alcoholism.... [T]he manifest functions of the policy of anonymity are indeed to protect the Fellowship and to affirm that the alcoholic is powerless, in Kurtz' words 'not-God.'"

In another, more recent example, Putnam (2000, p. 152), in his often-quoted study of declining civic participation, stated that groups such as AA do not add to social capital, because the individuals in them simply "focus on themselves in the presence of others." David Lewis (1999, p. 12), scholar and professor at Brown University, wrote that "the absence of effective community-based groups advocating the rights of and service for alcoholics and drug addicts is painfully obvious." He noted that the millions who have recovered through twelve-step programs make up a natural but "untapped" resource; members of such groups are "reluctant to come forward not only because of shame and humiliation, but also due to the anonymity principles of self-help." Taken together, these extraordinary statements show how little scholars in the alcoholism field understand the twelve-step community and its people.

In 2003a and b, L. F. Kurtz and M. Fisher explained that AA's eleventh tradition—"Our public relations policy is based on attraction rather than promotion; we need always maintain personal anonymity at the level of press, radio and film" (AA, 1976, p. 564)—recommends that members refrain from publicly announcing their connection to the fellowship. Anonymity is viewed within the fellowships as both a protection of confidentiality and a spiritual warning that protects members from the "corrupting influences of power, recognition, and public approval found in the world of politics" (as Beauchamp, 1980, p. 64, correctly stated). Beauchamp argued, however, that AA's anonymity tradition goes beyond the application to within-fellowship activity and represents a policy of secrecy.

It is true that AA and other fellowships (as a whole) are nonpolitical also because of their tenth tradition (traditions in other fellowships contain essentially the same wording): "Alcoholics Anonymous [or other twelve-step group] has no opinion on outside issues; hence the AA name ought never be drawn into public controversy" (AA, 1976, p. 564). The tenth tradition, however, aims only to prevent twelve-step participants from activity regarding outside issues "within" the fellowship or in the "name of the fellowship." It was not intended to prevent participation in civic and political activity outside the fellowship. (Can you imagine what would happen to AA if its membership began discussing the Affordable Care Act in meetings?) In reviewing the political impact of NCADD and placing it in its historical context, much social policy legislation on chemical dependency treatment and prevention can be traced to its activities, which were filled with people in twelve-step recovery programs (Brown & Brown, 2001; White, 1998).

Not only academics in the field misunderstand the recovering community's relationship with community service; the same is true of the average person. The first of the twelve steps—"We admitted we were powerless over alcohol, that our lives had become unmanageable" (AA, 1976, p. 59)—leads many to think that joining up with AA or another twelve-step group renders the participant completely powerless over his or her entire life and everything in it, even though the wording is "powerless over alcohol." For example, Williams (1992, p. 9) wrote about the admission of powerlessness that "a black person hears the call to powerlessness as one more command to lie down and take it." As pastor of Glide Memorial Church, he advocated a different way toward empowerment and sobriety. Another more recent example comes from the mental health advocacy movement:

> A common requirement in 12-step programs is to admit powerlessness and turn one's self and life over to the power and direction of a trusted *other* or Higher Power. While respecting the importance of spirituality for many people, in mental health recovery there is also emphasis on empowerment and self-determination—helping individuals to find their own voice and to take personal responsibility for their own lives. This is based on the belief that individuals need to reclaim, not turn over, their power as one of the first steps of a recovery process. (National Empowerment Center and the Recovery Consortium, 2007, p. 8)

A lack of understanding this very central principle of a twelve-step program is one reason many believe twelve-step fellowships are antithetical to the emergence of personal autonomy, empowerment, and community participation. This tendency to leap on some words without taking time to really understand them and their context has created an image of twelve-step members as reactionary and uninvolved in the life of the broader community. Nothing could be farther from the truth.

In 2003, Michael Fisher and I published findings from an investigation of the claim that twelve-step fellowships discouraged community involvement and advocacy (Kurtz & Fisher, 2003a, 2003b). We knew this was a myth because of what we saw going on all around us. Fisher is a community organizer in Detroit who develops programs that enhance neighborhoods, help the poor, and help people into recovery from substances. Many of his friends and fellow organizers affiliate with AA, NA, Alcoholics for Christ, and other such groups. We found a sample of thirty-three recovering individuals to interview with questions about how average participants in recovery programs felt about community involvement, how involved they were, and whether they had experienced discouragement or encouragement from fellow participants and the program as a whole.

Most of the NA participants came from the city of Detroit, and some were also members of Alcoholics for Christ. Their activities included such things as participation in neighborhood associations, block clubs, park cleanup committees, and a CB radio patrol—in other words, very grass-roots kinds of involvement. We found AA respondents in Ann Arbor and Toledo. They were more involved in established civic groups such as the Goodfellows, the Rotary Club, and the Chamber of Commerce than in local neighborhood groups. But both subgroups involved themselves in work with social service agencies by serving on boards and advisory committees and as employees involved in community organizing. Religious organizations, primarily churches, were the organizational context for an approximately equal number of AA and NA respondents. The numbers of organizations with which AA members affiliated ranged from one to ten, with a mean of 3.5 organizations per member. NA members' organizational affiliations ranged from one to nine, with a mean of 3.3.

Two AA respondents suggested that the key to community involvement was their sponsor. A forty-three-year-old African American AA female stated: "They told me don't drink, don't think, go to meetings, and get a sponsor. I did that. My sponsor said, 'You need to do community service,' and I did that." A sixty-three-year-old white male agreed that it was the sponsor who was the link to the community: "Instead of just answering questions, a sponsor should take them in hand and take them along on community service activities" (Kurtz & Fisher, 2003a, p. 895).

Many of our interview subjects thought they were empowered by learning skills that they needed in community work. Just being sober and clean enabled them to function in society after recovery and then to be open to serving the public when they saw service work modeled by other participants. Our subjects were not involved so much in a social movement as they were in giving back to the community that had given them a second chance after addiction. Only two of the thirty-three-member sample thought the traditions on anonymity deterred them from community service. For most, it was just the opposite, and twenty-five flatly rejected the idea. Most saw community service as an extension of twelfth-step work: "Having had a spiritual awakening as a result of these steps, we tried to carry this message to alcoholics and practice these principles in all our affairs" (AA, 1976, pp. 59–60).

Theoretically, twelve-step fellowships should be "empowering community settings" (Eastland, 1995; Kurtz & Fisher, 2003a). The fellowships provide opportunities for shared leadership, learning skills, participation in organizational tasks, and the development and reconstruction of new identities. Further, the twelve steps offer a belief system that involves reaching out to others and capitalizing on one's strengths. All of these facets have been identified as critical to the formation of empowerment. The activities we documented did not lead those in our sample to political action on a large scale or on the national level, such as the activities of the NCADD. But those days are coming.

RECOVERY COMMUNITY ORGANIZATIONS

A broad advocacy movement is building among recovering people, nationally and internationally. Although it had been there in an incipient form, the movement began organizationally in 2001, when a group of recovering people met in St. Paul, Minnesota, to plan for a national advocacy movement under the leadership of an organization they called Faces & Voices of Recovery (http://www.facesandvoicesofrecovery.org). A collection of recovering people had been planning for that meeting since the 1990s as a step toward forming an advocacy organization. The meeting in St. Paul became the Alliance Project; it subsequently planned a national gathering and a survey of the recovery community.

Out of this effort in 2001 came the Faces & Voices of Recovery Association of Recovery Community Organizations (ARCO), a network of local, regional, and statewide community organizations. The association assesses needs of people recovering from addictions, educates the public, creates community centers, and sponsors public events (recovery marches, rallies, concerts) that offer proof of the power of recovery (White, 2013). Local groups sponsor recovery walks to publicize and advocate for representation and voice for people in recovery and their family members at local, state, and federal policy levels. Recovery celebration events grew throughout the first decade of the twenty-first century from a handful of fledgling recovery marches that drew a few hundred people in 2000 to more than 125,000 recovering people and their families and friends participating in more than two hundred Recovery Month events during September 2010. Faces & Voices of Recovery provided central coordination of these events and has designated one event each year in a different city to be the national hub event.

ARCO has united and supported the network of local, regional, and statewide recovery organizations, linking them with local and national allies and providing training and technical assistance.

The Faces & Voices of Recovery mission in early 2014, according to the group's website, was as follows: 'Faces & Voices of Recovery is dedicated to organizing and mobilizing the over 20 million Americans in recovery from addiction to alcohol and other drugs, our families, friends and allies into recovery community organizations and networks, to promote the rights and resources to recover through advocacy, education and demonstrating the power and proof of long-term recovery."

Since its founding in 2001, this coalition has gained more than 25,000 members; it seeks to improve the lives of 43 million Americans affected by alcohol and other drugs through building the capacity of community organizations, to raise the profile of 20 million successfully recovering Americans, and to enhance recognition of peer recovery-support services. One undertaking has been the distribution of a documentary movie, *The Anonymous People.* It tells stories of recovery through the faces and voices of citizens, leaders, volunteers, corporate executives, public figures, and celebrities. Showings of the movie are arranged by local recovery groups, advertised locally, and presented in accessible public venues.

One of the state-level advocacy organizations affiliated with ARCO is PRO-A, the Pennsylvania Recovery Organization Alliance. This alliance of local organizations was established in 1998 to unite the state's recovery community. Its office is in Harrisburg, the state capital. The alliance works with regional organizations to develop organizational structure and help recovery groups in the state to work together. Its goals are to support quality services, combat stigma and discrimination, and represent the recovery community in Pennsylvania. ARCO events have also been joined by members of other addiction recovery mutual-aid groups listed on the Faces & Voices website (http://www.facesandvoicesofrecovery.org/guide/support).

As mentioned in chapter 2, the recovery advocacy movement has influenced national policy. The Office of National Drug Control Policy stated in its 2012 ONDCP Recovery Update that the key to reducing American's drug problem is greater support for and partnership with the millions of citizens who are in long-term recovery from addiction (http://www.whitehouse.gov/ondcp/recovery).

One of the challenges of the ARCO agenda will be to avoid powerful commercial interests that may offer funding in return for possible co-optation of the movement. The danger of this kind of usurpation has already been felt in the mental health arena, as will be seen in the next section.

NATIONAL ALLIANCE ON MENTAL ILLNESS

The National Alliance for the Mentally Ill (NAMI) began in Madison, Wisconsin, in 1979. A group of families of persons with mental illness hosted a conference and invited anyone with similar interests to attend. Two hundred eighty-four people representing fifty-nine family groups from twenty-nine states and Canada showed up, surprising the organizers. It was past time for such a group to form. "In three days they agreed on a name, purposes, and funding mechanisms; they drafted bylaws and selected a steering committee to bring the [organization] into existence" (Howe & Howe, 1987, p. 23). Nine months later, it was a tax-exempt legal entity with a Washington, D.C., office. In 1985, E. Fuller Torrey called it "the most important thing... since anti-psychotic drugs were introduced in the 1950s" (Howe & Howe, 1987, p. 24).

By the end of its sixth year, NAMI had grown to six hundred groups and was adding a new affiliate group every ten working hours. Families of people with serious mental illness had been observing the deinstitutionalization of state hospital patients during the previous twenty years, many of them ending up with one of those patients at home and not knowing how to cope with that. Families with newly diagnosed children struggled, unable to get treatment from a community mental health system that seemed to bypass the people who needed it most, while hospitals refused to admit people who were not yet a danger to themselves and others. In large numbers, they turned to NAMI affiliates springing up in towns and cities around the country. They compared notes and found that many of them had been told that they, the parents, had caused the disability wrecking their child's life. Together, they realized that they were all getting sold a "bill of goods."

In 1999, NAMI suffered a setback when criticism over its accepting donations from drug companies came out in *Mother Jones* magazine. That negative publicity continued for the next ten years. The concern was that NAMI's intense belief favoring psychiatric drugs as a necessary part of treatment may have been imposed on members by a national office supported by large donations from the pharmaceutical industry. In 2009, Senator Charles Grassley asked NAMI to reveal its support from the pharmaceutical industry, the implication being that the organization was a front for the trade and that it promoted drugs, some of questionable safety, to unsuspecting members. A long letter to NAMI membership from its executive director revealed that 56 percent of the budget came from pharmaceutical companies. In part, it said:

> NAMI's goal is to reduce the percentage of our budget that is supported by charitable donations from pharmaceutical companies. While we deeply appreciate the support we have received, we set this goal because we understand the value of diversifying our funding sources—both for fiscal stability and because we want to shed any lingering, unfair accusations that somehow NAMI has been "bought"—I can assure you: nothing could be further from the truth. NAMI's advocacy voice is loud and clear and uncompromised. http://www.mindfreedom.org/kb/psych-drug-corp/nami/nami-drug-companies

Today NAMI stands for National Alliance on Mental Illness, a name change that occurred around 2005. The organization has grown to 250,000 members, with more than 1,200 affiliated groups spanning all fifty states, the District of Columbia, Puerto Rico, and the Virgin Islands.

NAMI's best-known and most popular programs are found in its affiliate chapters, where local communities can refer people to NAMI-sponsored support groups, family education programs, membership meetings with speakers on topics relevant to psychiatric disability, and advocacy sponsorship locally, statewide, and nationally. Out of its central office, NAMI sponsored the program PACT Across America, a grass-roots effort to educate communities about assertive community treatment (ACT).

The PACT program involved developing a model ACT plan and manual, then disseminating the manual to state departments of mental health, state Medicaid offices, legislators, and others. NAMI members held workshops and presentations at the local level. At the national level, NAMI lobbyists pushed for congressional action to require states to provide ACT programs and pressured Medicare and Medicaid to pay for ACT services. ACT is an extensively researched and effective treatment intervention that provides intense treatment for people with serious mental disabilities, including efforts to increase independence and prevent homelessness and unnecessary hospitalization (Test & Stein, 1976).

Local affiliates sponsor public awareness programs and educational opportunities for families and the general public. Perhaps what NAMI is best known for at the local level are the support group programs for parents, siblings, and individuals with mental illness. In my community, NAMI sponsors support groups and a family education program for families who have a member with a psychiatric disability, and it publicizes other relevant supports in the community such as the local clubhouse, the consumer-run drop-in center, and the dual recovery group. In addition, eleven states have free six-week training courses for parents and other caregivers of individuals with mental illness. Some of these states offer courses in more than one city (Florida, Illinois, Missouri, North Carolina, and Virginia).

In 2003, an outside research firm surveyed a national randomly selected sample of 3,400 NAMI members in all fifty states (Hall, Graf, Fitzpatrick, Lane, & Birkel, 2003). The researchers found that most of the individuals with a psychiatric disorder were male, Caucasian, between the ages of eighteen and forty-four, unmarried, and living either alone or with their parents. They were poor; 71 percent lived on less than $20,000 a year, and one in five lived on less than $5,000 year. Income sources included SSDI (37 percent), SSI (35 percent), wages from a job (30 percent), and regular support from family members (19 percent). Slightly more than half had a high school education or less. Just more than two-thirds (67 percent) were unemployed.

Medicaid and Medicare were the primary forms of health insurance among individuals represented in the survey findings; 37 percent of respondents identified one or both as their form of health insurance coverage. Thirty-seven percent also relied on private health insurance, and 10 percent reported no health insurance coverage at all.

More than half (52 percent) of this group had diagnoses of schizophrenia, and 42 percent were diagnosed with bipolar disorder. Almost all of the respondents were on medication. Forty-four percent had been arrested at some point in their lives, and for 29 percent, the arrest had occurred in the past year; many did not receive appropriate treatment while incarcerated (Hall et al., 2003).

Additional responses and open-ended comments on survey response forms depicted dissatisfaction with and lack of access to services, public discrimination, and stigma so severe that it cost people their livelihood, ability to be employed without losing eligibility for disability payments and insurance coverage, and ability to afford to live independently. The results of the survey showed that the majority of people with mental health disabilities lacked the services needed to promote recovery, independence, and productivity. They lived with unacceptable barriers of stigma and discrimination stemming from failed public policy and the absence of effective services. The study's authors stated:

> From our perspective, one of the most unacceptable results from this survey concerns the chronic unemployment experienced by people with serious mental illnesses. Approximately two-thirds of individuals in our survey were unemployed.... According to the survey data, supported employment services were received by fewer than one-third of the individuals who needed it and, among those who received the service, access and quality were rated the poorest of all interventions. Obviously the implementation of quality supported employment services is scandalously lacking in the United States. (Hall et al., 2003, pp. 25–26)

After reading the report and considering the situation for people with serious psychiatric disabilities today, it's hard to see that any change has occurred in the ten years since its publication. One can hope that the recovery model of care driven by the President's New Freedom Commission on Mental Health in 2003 has begun to make productive changes at local levels and that NAMI on the national level will press for national policy action to make that happen (SAMHSA, 2003).

Since the report came out, NAMI has launched a treatment and recovery information and advocacy database (TRIAD) for the purpose of collecting data that characterize the gap between the services, supports, and environment necessary for recovery and what actually exists in each state. This will be used to inform advocacy efforts with better data to achieve better services (http://www.nami.org).

In 2009, NAMI's national office produced a fifty-one-page brochure entitled *Reinvesting in the Community: A Family Guide to Expanding Home and Community-Based Mental Health Services and Supports.* This document describes the existing residential supports for children with mental illness and explains many of the drawbacks of the existing system of care, or noncare in some cases, and defines needed changes that will allow children to be treated at or near home. NAMI intends this publication's extensive information to assist local chapters in advocating for supports in local areas. One of the supports described is a Medicaid waiver program, which allows states the ability to use Medicaid for services not normally covered; the waiver has been adopted in three states (Kansas, Michigan, New York) with good results (Gruttadaro, Markey, & Duckworth, 2009). This publication is an example of the work that NAMI's national staff produces and passes on to states and local affiliates.

NAMI remains the most well-known and ubiquitous advocacy association for mental health conditions in the United States; however, there are many others, and many of those have a different philosophical and practical approach to mental health conditions and their causes and treatments. These can be grouped under the heading of consumer/survivor organizations.

CONSUMER/SURVIVOR ORGANIZATIONS

Advocacy in the modern mental health field goes back to 1908, when Clifford Beers published his classic autobiography *A Mind That Found Itself.* In it, he tells of a three-year period during which he was psychotic, his healthy mind lost and then regained. His story reveals the condition of "insane asylums" of the period. Beers went on to found the Mental Hygiene Movement which created the Mental Health Association, now called Mental Health America. MHA is a lobbying, advocacy, and public education association that has been working through its local affiliates for more than one hundred years to advocate for changes in mental health policy and to educate the public (http://www.mentalhealthamerica.net/about-us). MHA members include recovering people, mental health professionals, and interested supporters from all walks of life.

Psychiatric survivor groups have evolved from the mental patients liberation movement of the 1970s. They exist in almost every state, especially California, Ohio,

Maryland, Vermont, Florida, Kentucky, Massachusetts, and Oregon (National Empowerment Center and Recovery Consortium, 2007). These groups represent considerable diversity of opinion about mental illness, particularly when contrasted with the unified voices of NAMI. Many consumer/survivors have recovered from the mental illness they experienced initially, many are less or not at all dependent on psychotropic medications, and most oppose involuntary treatments of any kind, especially those that involve electroconvulsive therapy and isolation rooms. Some regard many of the drugs given to people with mental health conditions as a form of pharmaceutical lobotomy and cite research that suggests the drugs damage the frontal lobe of the brain. Some survivor groups don't believe in psychiatric labels, and members prefer not to think of themselves as having a mental illness.

The consumer movement began with ex-patients coming together as a civil rights crusade in the 1970s and the development of groups such as the Oregon Insane Liberation Front, thought to be the first consumer-run rights group for mental patients (Tomes, 2006). Inspired by civil rights struggles of African Americans, women, and gay pride, they celebrated "mad pride." As mentioned in chapter 2, Judi Chamberlin's 1978 book, *On Our Own: Patient Controlled Alternatives to the Mental Health System*, heralded the philosophy and direction of the movement toward patients having a say both in their treatment and in the organizations themselves (Tomes, 2006). The more radical groups, such as the National Association of Mental Patients, espoused using the term "survivor," whereas the moderate National Association of Mental Health Consumers preferred the term "consumer," so the merged appellation "consumer/survivor movement" caught on.

Some take issue with the combined terminology by saying that the two terms convey very different meanings (Sharfstein & Dickerson, 2006). The consumer groups have had a major impact on how mental health services are delivered. Consumers use services. Those who think of themselves as survivors of the mental health system are a vocal and small minority of ex-patients who claim to be victims of harsh treatment, such as involuntary hospitalization, isolation rooms, and electroconvulsive therapy. Some deny that mental illness exists (Sharfstein & Dickerson, 2006, p. 734). Less radical and more willing to work with the psychiatric establishment, consumer groups have grown and influenced policy, whereas survivor groups have become less significant according to this point of view.

In response to pressure from patient and ex-patient groups, the federal government began funding conferences for consumer groups in 1980 (Frese & Davis, 1997). In 1992, the Center for Mental Health Services funded the National Mental Health Consumers' Self-Help Clearinghouse in Philadelphia and the National Empowerment Center in Lawrence, Massachusetts. Consumers also influenced the development of the Center for Psychiatric Rehabilitation at Boston University.

Today federal law requires that states receiving funds for mental health services must have consumers on all mental health boards. Another important outcome of the consumer movement has been the development of peer-support specialist credentialing, training, and inclusion among the staff of mental health centers.

The National Coalition for Mental Health Recovery was formed in 2006. Today it represents thirty-six member organizations (thirty-two states and four national technical assistance centers). To join the coalition, a group must be consumer/survivor-run (that is, the majority of the board and the staff are consumers/survivors), it must be involved with consumers/survivors statewide or in a significant region of the state, and it must be inclusive and representative of the state. The organization's board must approve in writing the mission and statement of purpose itself and any other organization. The voice of consumers/survivors must be central to decision-making at all levels (Fisher & Spiro, 2010).

Some of the more radical survivor groups have been taken over by larger organizations, such as the Church of Scientology. One that has not been co-opted is MindFreedom International. According to its website (http://www.mindfreedom.org), MindFreedom is one of the very few totally independent groups in the mental health field, having no funding from or control by governments, drug companies, religions, corporations, or the mental health system. Also, one reads on the website that the majority of MindFreedom's members include people who have experienced human rights violations in the mental health system, mental health professionals and workers, advocates and attorneys, family members, and the general public. Any of these can be active as equal members and leaders in the MindFreedom International community.

David Oakes, who cofounded MindFreedom International in 1986, is a good example of those involved in the survivor movement. When he was a student at Harvard in the mid-1970s, Oakes experienced several symptoms that seemed to warrant psychiatric treatment. This treatment included episodes of solitary confinement and forced drugging with tranquilizers. Doctors told him he would have to take the drugs for the rest of his life, that he was seriously mentally ill and would stay that way. Although hospitalized five times during that period, Oakes continued his studies at Harvard. His academic program placed him in an internship with Mental Patients Liberation Front, which met at Vocations for Social Change near Central Square in Cambridge, Massachusetts. According to his biographical sketch on the MindFreedom website, "David wrote his senior paper about this experience of community organizing with psychiatric survivors, and graduated with honors in 1977.... It was while in a psychiatric solitary confinement cell in Bowditch Hall in McLean Hospital in Belmont, Massachusetts, that David decided he wanted, once freed, to take action to improve the mental health system" (http://www.mindfreedom.org/who-we-are/david-w-oaks). He discontinued taking drugs and has remained drug- and symptom-free since 1977. Since then, his life has been devoted to rights for mental patients and the environmental, peace, and social justice movements. Oakes was the executive director of MindFreedom International until December 2012, when he fell and severed his spinal cord. His progress in recovery from this devastating injury is described on his personal website (www.davidwoakes.com).

MindFreedom International is a coalition of one hundred grass-roots and affiliate groups throughout the nation and around the world seeking rights for people labeled with psychiatric disabilities. As such, it joins other advocacy groups for mental health and psychiatric survivor networks around the country and internationally. Its goals are (1) to win human rights campaigns in mental health, (2) to challenge abuse by the psychiatric drug industry, (3) to support the self-determination of psychiatric survivors and mental health consumers, and (4) to promote safe, humane, and effective options in mental health.

CONCLUSION

Both the mental health and the addiction treatment fields are in early stages of developing advocacy networks. The addiction network is potentially larger because of its armies of "anonymous" people. Another difference between the mental health consumer groups and the network of recovering people existing in the social world of twelve-step fellowships is that the majority of the former receive government funding, whereas Anonymous groups do not. Ex-mental patients and current mental health consumers have a thirty-six-year history of organizing and advocating for change and have gotten the attention of policy makers in Washington. The anonymous people have yet to achieve the same degree of support.

The next chapter is about three forms of service delivery that include varying degrees of help with employment, housing, and mutual help. All three involve peer-support staff as integral to the running of the programs, and all three are relatively free from dependence on government funding.

REFERENCES

AA. (1955). *Alcoholics Anonymous: The story of how many thousands of men and women have recovered from alcoholism* (2nd ed.). New York, NY: AA World Services.

AA. (1976). *Alcoholics Anonymous: The story of how many thousands of men and women have recovered from alcoholism* (3rd ed.). New York, NY: AA World Services.

Beauchamp, D. E. (1980). *Beyond alcoholism: Alcohol and public health policy*. Philadelphia, PA: Temple University Press.

Beers, C. (1908/1923). *A mind that found itself*. Garden City, NY: Doubleday.

Brown, S., & Brown, D. R. (2001). *Mrs. Marty Mann: The first lady of Alcoholics Anonymous*. Center City, MN: Hazelden.

Chamberlin, J. (1978). *On our own: Patient controlled alternatives to the mental health system*. New York, NY: Hawthorn Books.

Eastland, L. S. (1995). Recovery as an interactive process: Explanation and empowerment in 12-step programs. *Qualitative Health Research, 5*(3), 292–314.

Fisher, D., & Spiro, L. (2010). Finding and using our voice: How consumer/survivor advocacy is transforming mental health care. In L. D. Brown & S. Wituk (Eds.), *Mental health self-help*. New York, NY: Springer.

Frese, F. J., & Davis, W.W. (1997). The consumer-survivor movement, recovery, and consumer professionals. *Professional Psychology Research and Practice, 28*(3), 243–245.

Gruttadaro, D., Markey, D., & Duckworth, K. (2009). *Reinvesting in the community: A family guide to expanding home and community-based mental health services and supports*. Arlington, VA: NAMI. Available at http://www.nami.org/Content/NavigationMenu/NAMILand/CAACricguide.pdf

Hall, L. A., Graf, A. C., Fitzpatrick, M. J., Lane, T., & Birkel, R. C. (2003). *Shattered lives: Results of a national survey of NAMI members and their families*. Available at http://goo.gl/722h8z

Howe, C. W., & Howe, J. W. (1987). The National Alliance for the Mentally Ill: History and ideology. In A. Hatfield (Ed.), *Families of the mentally ill: Meeting the challenges* (pp. 23–33). San Francisco, CA: Jossey-Bass.

Kurtz, L. F., & Fisher, M. (2003a). Participation in community life by AA and NA members. *Contemporary Drug Problems, 30*(Winter), 875–904.

Kurtz, L. F., & Fisher, M. (2003b). Twelve-step recovery and community service. *Health and Social Work, 28*(2), 137–145.

Lewis, D. L. (1999). Advocacy and 12-step anonymity. *Brown University Digest of Addiction Theory and Application, 18*(2), 12.

National Empowerment Center and Recovery Consortium. (2007). *Voices of transformation: Developing recovery-based statewide consumer/survivor organizations*. Retrieved from http://www.power2u.org/downloads/Voices%20of%20Transformation.pdf

Putnam, R. D. (2000). *Bowling alone: The collapse and revival of American community*. New York, NY: Simon & Shuster.

SAMHSA. (2003). *New Freedom Commission on Mental Health, achieving the promise: Transforming mental health care in America*. Final report. (DHHS Publication No. SMA-03-3832. Rockville, MD.) Available at www.mentalhealthcommission.gov

Sharfstein, S. S., & Dickerson, F. B. (2006). Psychiatry and the consumer movement. *Health Affairs, 25*(3), 734–736.

Test, M. A., & Stein, L. I. (1976). Practical guidelines for the community treatment of markedly impaired patients. *Community Mental Health Journal, 12*, 72–82.

Tomes, N. (2006). The patient as a policy factor: A historical case study of the consumer/survivor movement. *Health Affairs, 25*(3), 720–729.

White, W. L. (1998). *Slaying the dragon: A history of addiction treatment and recovery in America*. Bloomington, IL: Lighthouse Institute.

White, W. L. (2010). Today we stand. PRO-ACT Recovery Walks 2010 National Rally for Recovery Site, September 25, 2010. Philadelphia, PA. Available from http://www.williamwhitepapers.com/papers

White, W. L. (2013). State of the new recovery advocacy movement. Amplification of remarks to the Association of Recovery Community Organizations at Faces & Voices of Recovery Executive Directors Leadership Academy. Dallas, TX, November 15. Available from http://www.williamwhitepapers.com/papers

Williams, C. (1992). *No hiding place: Empowerment and recovery for our troubled communities.* New York, NY: HarperCollins.

[T]hey will only succeed if they can operate their own programs.
FAIRWEATHER (1994, p. 70)

12

HOUSING, EMPLOYMENT, AND MUTUAL HELP

RECOVERING PEOPLE NEED at least three things: shelter, work, and supportive peer relationships. This chapter shows how the self-help mutual-aid philosophy and movement have influenced the development of formal program models in the mental health and addiction services sectors. Three model programs provide for all three of these needs: Fairweather Lodges, Oxford Houses, and Fountain House. In all three, mutual support is central to the method, and all three types of programs have shown remarkable success when implemented. For too many people with mental health conditions, addictions, or both, social isolation is all they have unless they are in jail. Effective programs are in short supply, and there is no good reason for that. None of the three programs discussed here is new; all have been around for at least thirty-eight years, the oldest for sixty-five years.

FAIRWEATHER LODGES

Founder

George Fairweather came to the same conclusion neuropsychiatrist Abraham Low did: no amount of inpatient treatment could overcome the sabotaging effects of community stigma focused on the patients he discharged. Low started Recovery, Inc., intending it to be a pressure group to change his state's commitment law, which he blamed for the indignities his discharged patients encountered (Low, 1943/1991). He was unsuccessful, but even if the law had changed, the stigma would have remained. Twenty-six years later, Fairweather found that successful treatment on an inpatient treatment unit did not carry over after discharge; ex-patients relapsed in the face of discrimination and lack of group supports (Fairweather,

1994). Fairweather, a young Ph.D. psychologist in the 1950s, worked in an inpatient program in Palo Alto, California (Fairweather, 1994; Fairweather, Sanders, Maynard, & Cressler, 1969). This was just before deinstitutionalization became public mental health policy, a time when patients stayed in mental hospitals for years or left and reentered often. By examining aftercare statistics, Fairweather learned that 75 percent of discharged patients returned to the hospital even though they had been released as "cured" or "much improved" (Fairweather, 1994, p. 44). In 1963, he developed a community program for ex-patients that gave them the support he hoped would allow them to succeed after discharge. The program he invented came to be known as Fairweather Lodges. It combined group support, housing, and employment in one package.

Founding Story

Fairweather's initial effort was to set up inpatient problem-solving groups in which the patients together would solve their mental health problems, while the staff stood by and consulted when asked. His earlier research led him to think that the groups would work only if certain conditions existed: (1) leadership came from within the group, (2) members received meaningful rewards, (3) leadership was good leadership, and (4) members perceived the group as helpful to them (Fairweather, 1980, p. 9). He designed a plan, implemented it, and studied outcomes. He believed that the group process would provide members with needed skills and emotional support to sustain them in the community.

His plan worked well while patients were still in the hospital, but once they returned to the community, they continued to relapse and reenter the inpatient ward. Returning patients reported that they needed the support of a group to help them through hard times with their symptoms and with the community's rejection. Further, they needed housing and employment, which were scarce.

This led Fairweather to his experimental community venture, which he refers to as a small-group society project. He found an old motel with a kitchen and enough rooms to house an entire ward of twenty-five men, most with psychotic diagnoses. They were simultaneously discharged, with a plan to live together and form a business in which they could work and earn income. The daring plan worked; the old motel became the first Fairweather Lodge. With Fairweather's help and consultation from a janitorial coach, they established a cleaning service, where some members acted as crew chiefs and each had a job doing whatever he was able to do in the new business. The group's experience in problem solving on the hospital ward had prepared the members to establish rules and procedures for dealing with psychiatric symptoms, lapses in judgment, and work habits outside. Over time, the business became successful and financially rewarding for some, but not all, of the members (Fairweather, 1994).

Fairweather believed that the small-group process used in running the lodge by the ex-patients should be learned while they were still in the hospital. For this reason, he directed that patients going into the community together should be from the same hospital ward. Lodge principles state that "peer support is ultimately more powerful than assistance from paid service providers" (http://www.theccl.org/FairweatherLodge/Standards.aspx). They met together four days a week, progressing through steps in which they solved problems about how they would manage once they left the hospital for group living in the community. Patients volunteered for the experimental condition and then were matched with other patients who did not volunteer and who, therefore, constituted a comparison group for research purposes. Following the introduction of the first lodge, additional lodges began forming in other parts of the country, helped along by staff from the first experiment.

Program Today

In 1978, administrators and staff of existing lodges around the country formed the Coalition for Community Living to promote community support systems and educate the public about Fairweather Lodges. The coalition also engages in research and provides information to care providers. Its website (http://www.theccl.org) describes the program's principles, practices, and outcome measures and provides links to lodges throughout the country. Lodges serve both men and women, and some provide services for women with children.

As described on the website, Fairweather Lodges begin with a group of hospital patients who volunteer to become lodge members. These patients divide into groups whose members vary in skills and capabilities. Groups elect leaders and work together to develop problem-solving abilities. The goal of the group is to utilize the small-group problem-solving process to generate solutions to any problem they face. This type of group work helps individuals complete their treatment programs more quickly than they would do otherwise, and the ability to solve problems together is crucial to the group's survival as a working lodge in the community.

> Typically lodges are small groups of 4 to 8 people who share a house and own a small business. Each group must select a business to operate, for which they will develop and implement a business plan. Lodge groups' businesses have included lawn care, custodial or laundry services, printing, furniture building, shoe repair, catering, and other services. Lodge members assume specific positions of responsibility within the household and the business; for example,

> the business may have a manager and crew chief; the household, a cook and a medication supervisor. There is no live-in staff at any Lodge, although each Lodge has access to a professional who is available for training and consultation whenever the group requests his or her help. Staff members are also on call 24 hours a day for emergencies. In addition, Lodge members hire professional consultants—such as accountants and lawyers—to assist with Lodge business operations. Responsibility for the house and business improves the members' self-confidence and helps them become more independent than they would normally be by giving them a stable role in the community. (http://www.theccl.org/FairweatherLodge.aspx#sec3)

The original lodge had thirteen principles; that list has now been reduced to eight (see box 12.1). Added to the eight principles are sixteen required practices that lead to sixteen outcome measures, all of which can be found in detail on the website. "A comprehensive assessment of Lodge success, therefore, involves: (1) Adherence to the Lodge Principles; (2) Implementation of Lodge Practices; (3) Demonstrated

BOX 12.1

EIGHT PRINCIPLES OF THE FAIRWEATHER LODGE MODEL

1. The lodge must provide a safe, healthy and caring environment, which reinforces the recovery process.
2. The lodge must be a part of the plan for managing symptoms and promoting good mental health.
3. Services must be available as long as the participant wants and needs them.
4. People with psychiatric disabilities increase their community success and raise their social status through employment, through accumulating wealth and through direct consumerism. Opportunities for promotion and rising to a higher status are provided.
5. Above and beyond economic roles, participants need to have meaningful roles in both the lodge and the larger community.
6. A successful lodge resembles a healthy family.
7. In order to progress, people with psychiatric disabilities need autonomy commensurate with their behavioral abilities, with the ultimate goal of full autonomy. The program must provide the consumers as much autonomy as possible.
8. Lodges must not be dependent on resources from any single entity.

---

http://theccl.org/FairweatherLodge/Standards.aspx

Outcomes; and (4) Participant Satisfaction" (http://theccl.org/FairweatherLodge/Standards.aspx). The coalition certifies successful lodges.

Financing

The first Fairweather Lodge project was supported by a federal grant to Stanford University. This was in conjunction with a nonprofit rehabilitation agency that had existing agreements with local labor unions and industries defining the workers as involved in rehabilitation and thereby excluded from union-management work contracts. Research and treatment staff salaries came from the grant, which also supplemented costs of running the lodge. By the end of the five-year research period, Fairweather was unable to find any agency, including the nonprofit rehabilitation agency, that would adopt the program and help defray its costs. For this reason, the initial lodge had to become completely self-supporting. This resulted in sixteen residents leaving the lodge because they could not or would not pay enough for their care; the other nine remained and became self-sufficient by operating the janitorial business (Fairweather et al., 1969). Most of the residents who left the lodge returned to the hospital.

Lodges now receive a mix of funding through community mental health budgets, from vocational rehabilitation grants to residents, donations, and self-funding from lodge businesses, and also from payments directly by residents, some of whom receive social security disability payments. Lodge practices require that programs not be dependent on resources from any single entity.

The lodges that followed the original were not successful in becoming self-sufficient through the businesses they started. This was one of the problems encountered by the hospital units that attempted to adopt the lodge concept; they had to compete with other hospital and mental health center programs for scarce funds. Despite the success of lodges in keeping people out of a hospital, they have not been part of hospital established structure. In addition, lodges have had to deal with governmental accreditation standards, local zoning laws, and traditional group home licensing. All of this requires investment by lodge administration staff (Mateer, 1980).

Diffusion

In 1980, Fairweather and his associates at Michigan State University published a twenty-five-year retrospective detailing their efforts to disseminate the lodge idea. Researchers traced their efforts from the date when the lodge research began on the hospital ward, around 1955. Beginning in 1967, Fairweather and fellow researchers contacted all 263 mental hospitals in the nation, asking them to consider learning about and possibly initiating lodge groups for patients ready for discharge. Only 5 percent agreed to establish a lodge society. Of those, "twenty-five hospitals were eventually persuaded to adopt the Lodge society" (Fairweather, 1980, p. 38). Six of those, by the end of five years, had adopted thirty separate lodges (Fergus, 1980).

This led to a second nationwide attempt to disseminate the lodge concept through contacts with hospitals and offers to do on-site training. By the end of 1978, there were thirty-four "adopters" (Fergus, 1980, p. 49). Michigan State psychologists had by then set up the Coalition for Community Living, made up of representatives from lodge programs whose purpose was to disseminate the lodge concept. Although the coalition still exists, the researchers found that it was difficult for representatives to allocate time and energy to its work, because their job of keeping their own lodges going and funded was so extensive and time-consuming.

Fairweather's success with his small-group society project did not result in wholesale revamping of community mental health programs, but his model slowly spread around the country in the fifty years since the first lodge began. Today there are ninety Fairweather Lodges in sixteen states (http://www.theccl.org/FairweatherLodge.aspx). The book containing the twenty-five-year retrospective includes descriptions of four lodge programs in different parts of the country. Of those four, only one still exists, in Hot Springs, Arkansas.

Success Rates

During the five years of the small-group society research project, Fairweather measured progress, such as number of returns to a hospital, behavioral improvements, and costs, which he contrasted with outcomes of traditional community programs (Fairweather et al., 1969; Fairweather, 1994). On every measure, his experimental program came out ahead. For example, only 5 percent of his men had been rehospitalized, compared with 75 percent of those in other programs. All of the small-group members worked two-thirds of the time, whereas most of those in other programs remained unemployed.

The Coalition for Community Living does not measure success for individual houses in the program. Programs have their own systems in place to measure accomplishment. These typically show decreases in hospitalizations for psychiatric symptoms, an increase in self-worth and confidence of individuals participating in the programs, increases in the length of time working in the community, and increases in skill (http://www.theccl.org/FAQ.aspx#q2). The Fairweather Lodges have been successful in providing housing and mutual support but only partially successful in providing employment for residents.

OXFORD HOUSES

Founder

In 1975, J. Paul Molloy became the founder of one of country's most successful community programs for addicts, which he called Oxford House. His story is told in a 2008 book, *Rescued Lives: The Oxford House Approach to Substance Abuse*, by a group of researchers at DePaul University in Chicago (Jason, Olson, & Foli, 2008). Molloy started drinking alcohol in college. He continued to drink as he finished law school and worked for a US Senator from Vermont, Winston Prouty, in Washington, DC. Eventually, he became the Republican counsel to the Senate Finance Committee, but his life was in shambles. He was drinking two fifths a day. His wife left him; he entered a psychiatric hospital, spent some time on the street, then entered a twenty-eight-day substance abuse program and finally a halfway house. By this time, Molloy was attending AA meetings. When the halfway house closed as a result of loss of funding, an AA member helped Molloy and other residents of the house pay the rent and take it over themselves.

Founding Story

The new residents of the house had no funds to hire staff, so they decided to form a democratic management among themselves. They called the home Oxford House after the Oxford Groups, a religious movement that inspired the beginnings of AA. The first house was in Silver Spring, Maryland, where the group's World Service Office continues with administrative authority. Soon after the first house opened, beds were filled, and more people asked for admission. This led the residents to open another house and, not long after that, a third. From 1975 to 1987, thirteen houses opened in the Washington area.

Expansion was slow until 1988. In that year, the Anti-Drug Abuse Act of 1988 passed and included a provision that required states that received federal block grants for alcoholism, drug addiction, or mental illness to set up a $100,000 revolving loan fund through which groups of six or more recovering people could borrow up to $4,000 to rent a house (White, 2012). Thirteen states allocate funds to hire recruiters to help set up the houses; when one house fills up, another is established. All recruiters are former Oxford House residents.

Program Today

An Oxford House has no time limit on how long a resident can remain, and this is important, because some people need extensive support over a long period to attain stable sobriety. The charter for an Oxford House requires the following: (1) it must be democratically self-run and follow policies and procedures determined by the residents of the house, (2) it must be financially self-supporting, and (3) it must expel any resident who returns to use of alcohol or illicit drugs. Its program is simple. Residents live together, share tasks in keeping up the house, work, pay rent, and attend AA or other self-help mutual-aid groups in the community. Oxford House, Inc., stands behind individual houses by giving those who apply and meet requirements a charter. Although it cannot guarantee a landlord that the residents will pay the rent, it does maintain regular contact with the house to make certain it is run in a responsible manner (Oxford House, 2011).

All Oxford Houses are rented ordinary single-family houses in good neighborhoods. There are houses for men and women with children, but there are no coed houses. The average number of residents per house is about eight, with a range of six to sixteen (Jason et al., 2008).

Financing

All Oxford Houses are autonomous and self-governing, which greatly reduces the cost of service. New houses begin with a start-up loan of $4,000 from the Oxford House World Services Office or a local government source. The house repays this loan at the rate of $170 a month for twenty-four months. This permits the house to pay the first month's rent and security deposit. Oxford Houses, in general, need at least seven residents so that the amount each person pays for rent and other expenses is not more than he or she can afford, although some houses have fewer occupants. Most tenants work and contribute about $100 a month toward an average of $1,380 rent. Houses are located in neighborhoods with low crime rates, which helps residents stay away from trouble spots (Oxford House, 2012). Other expenses are for recruiters who work for the World Service Office and travel to establish new homes, where they stay for short periods to assist. These costs are borne by state governments in some cases and by the Oxford House World Service Office in others. The central office raises funds through donations, grants, and contributions from the existing homes. Oxford Houses are cost-effective. Residents receive help in finding employment.

Diffusion

After passage of the Anti-Drug Abuse Act of 1988 which allocated funds for recruitment, growth of Oxford Houses exploded; as of 2013, recruiters have opened 1,612 Oxford Houses, providing 12,735 recovery beds in forty-five states; there are also 42 houses in four foreign countries (Canada, United Kingdom, Ghana, and Australia). Oxford House, Inc., employs a staff of seventy-three (in

2012), most of whom are recruiters (White, 2012). Oxford House, Inc., is an independent, public, nonprofit 501(c)(3) corporation that receives funds from contributions by the houses, from United Way and similar charities, and from states that pay for recruiters. The Oxford House website describes the World Council as follows:

> The World Council is comprised of 12 members: 9 of which presently live in an Oxford House, and 3 alumni. Members are elected each year at the Oxford House World Convention. The primary mission of the Oxford House World Council is to facilitate adherence to Oxford House Traditions' concept and system of operations, by providing effective means of communication and mission focus between the various organizational structures of Oxford House as a whole. In carrying out its mission the Council always keeps the focus on expansion of the network of individual Oxford Houses, to provide all recovering alcoholics and drug addicts the opportunity to develop comfortable sobriety without relapse. (http://www.oxfordhouse.org/userfiles/file/purpose_and_structure.php#structure)

The board of directors maintains the sole right to charter and to revoke the charter of individual Oxford Houses. It also exercises authority over the policies and officers of Oxford House, Inc. In this way, Oxford House, Inc., remains responsive to the needs of the population it serves (Oxford House, 2011). Oxford Houses are considered single-family residences for the purpose of zoning. Amendments to the 1988 Federal Fair Housing Act make it unlawful for any jurisdiction to discriminate against congregate living for the disabled (Jason et al., 2008; Oxford House, 2011). This law has made it possible for houses to open and operate in good neighborhoods with low crime rates, near shopping outlets, and away from bars, drug dealers, and prostitutes.

Success Rates

Longitudinal research by psychologists at DePaul University provides evidence that the Oxford House program is "successful, simple, and inexpensive" (Jason, et al., 2008, p. 178). Abstinence rates among residents have been 69 to 87 percent. One study followed nine hundred residents in 213 houses in sixteen states for one year, with interviews every four months. They found a relapse rate of 13.5 percent for those currently in houses and 18.5 percent for those who had left the house. About 65percent of residents cycle out of the house after a year; those who spend at least six months in residence have increased self-efficacy and abstinence.

Another study reported by the same authors (Jason, et al., 2008) followed residents of Oxford Houses in Illinois and compared them with the same number of residents randomly assigned to alternative living situations, all after undergoing treatment for addiction. The study lasted for twenty-four months. The findings showed that 69 percent of the Oxford House residents refrained from substance use, contrasted with 35 percent of the comparison group. Oxford House residents also experienced higher net incomes and lower incarceration rates than those who lived in different quarters (own home, relative's home, staffed recovery home, home of a spouse, homeless shelter, substance abuse treatment setting, home of a friend).

In an interview in 2012, Paul Molloy said:

> even with an annual turnover rate of 2.1, the Oxford House recovery bed inventory serves only about 26,000 recovering individuals each year or only a small percentage of the number who would benefit from living in an Oxford House. According to the federal government, about 2.3 million of the 25 million with an addiction to alcohol or other drugs received treatment last year—less than one in ten. Of those in formal treatment, sixty percent had been in treatment at least three times before their present treatment episode. Cycling in and out of treatment is the norm. Neither afflicted individuals nor society at large can afford that kind of inefficiency. (White, 2012, p. 17)

FOUNTAIN HOUSE

Founder

Although the clubhouse first came into being in the mid-1940s, when We Are Not Alone (WANA), the small self-help group, rented the building, it was really John Beard who developed the program that we think of today as the clubhouse model. Beard began his social work career at Wayne County General Hospital in Detroit, where he was first a student doing an internship and later a staff social worker. He and two colleagues developed a method of task-centered group work called Activity Group Therapy (AGT), which was based on their hypothesis that people with schizophrenia retained an ability to work and that if patients were encouraged to complete tasks, their mental condition would improve (Doyle, Lanoil, & Dudek, 2013). Experiments with this method were successful. As early as the mid-1950s, Beard and his colleagues had conceived of an intervention based on patient strengths rather than symptoms. It would be about forty years before the rest of the social work profession discovered the strengths approach (Rapp & Goscha, 2012).

Beard left Detroit to take a position at Fountain House in 1955. What he found when he got there was a settlement-house-like program with members of WANA in conflict with the board of directors and the staff. Beard wanted to redirect the program to use what he had learned in Detroit. It took him a year before he was able to modify the program into what would become the clubhouse model we know today, an amalgam of AGT and milieu therapy that harked back to methods of eighteenth-century moral treatment (Doyle et al., 2013).

Founding Story

Fountain House began at Rockland State Hospital in Orangeburg, New York, just north of New York City. It was at Rockland State in 1939 that the newly formed AA fellowship held its first "institutional" meetings in a mental hospital for the purpose of serving the alcoholics being treated there (http://www.aaseny.org/archives/history_book/rockland.pdf). Hiram Johnson, M.D., the psychiatrist on the ward, was impressed with AA and wanted to apply the same concept of self-help to patients on a psychiatric ward. He, together with a wealthy staff member, Elizabeth Schermerhorn, began a self-help fellowship for mental patients in the Male Reception Building in early 1943 (Anderson, 1998). Patients in this ward were known for their relapses and returns to the hospital, which prompted the effort to form a group to prepare patients for discharge. The idea was to have the patients form friendships that would follow them after discharge and somewhat protect them when faced with stigma and discrimination in the community.

After discharge, one of the patients contacted Schermerhorn about his idea for continuing to visit Rockland State in order to form a fellowship for former patients. This group began meeting and adopted the name We Are Not Alone (WANA) in 1944. An outside board of directors, including YMCA supporters, formed to provide access to needed resources. In spring of 1948, these supporters found a brownstone on West 47th Street in Manhattan with a fountain on the patio. In June 1948, the board of directors formed the Fountain House Foundation, Inc. (Anderson, 1998). The self-help group WANA also formed a management group, which they called the Fountain House Fellowship in order to preserve the self-help character of the clubhouse. In time, WANA as a separate group faded away, but the fellowship began offering social and recreational activities on evenings and weekends. By 1949, the house had received federal funding that was used to hire professional staff, including a professional executive director. The state's Department of Vocational Rehabilitation provided additional funds to set up training courses. The executive director meanwhile wanted to start providing therapy for members, which embroiled her in a controversy that led to her resignation.

A subsequent director soon found the program entangled in more conflict over the direction of the program, who would control the fellowship, and what activities would take place. Faced with the problems that the building had become too small for the larger numbers of ex-patients who applied for membership and tight funds, she resigned. A third director attempted to gain power amid conflicts involving almost every committee, board, and group associated with Fountain House. Despite this situation, the current program retains some of the original features: specifically, its focus on employment through vocational rehabilitation, the fact that involvement means membership rather than patient status, and efforts to preserve a self-help philosophy.

In early 1955, Beard dropped by Fountain House on his way to a conference and met Schermerhorn and others. The board had designed a new position of field director to organize mental patients in various parts of New York City. Beard seemed to be a good fit for that role, but it took several months for Schermerhorn to persuade him to move to New York in order to join the staff (Anderson, 1998). Later in 1955, the third director was asked to resign, and Beard became executive director. After a year, the fellowship board was eliminated as a result of ongoing agitation and divisiveness.

For the rest of his time as director, Beard developed Fountain House into the working community model it is today. He first developed the work units within the house and then transitional employment placements for those ready to work outside the house. Social and recreational activities were scheduled in the evenings, weekends, and holidays. By 1961, Fountain House had eight apartments for lease to members, two to an apartment, and the numbers in housing continued to grow. Beard served as director for twenty-seven years until his death in 1982 at the age of fifty-nine.

Program Today

Fountain House today occupies a different building (built in 1965) on West 47th Street, along with six brownstones to the west of the main building, a wellness center in the building, HUD-funded supportive housing throughout the city, a medical care storefront, the Sidney Baer Center on West 37th Street, and a farm in New Jersey. In 1976, Fountain House was awarded an NIMH grant to establish a national training program to teach the model to community-based organizations.

> Today members and staff collaborate on research, training, a wellness center, education, horticulture, full-time employment, intake, and orientation. Fountain House also incorporates a number of other work areas such as

> accounting, fundraising, human resources, and maintenance, which sustain its administration as an independent social agency.... Fountain House has expanded its scope to include an international training institute and a member art gallery. (Doyle et al., 2013, pp. 40–41)

Its founders described Fountain House as an intentional community with four important messages for everyone who chose to become involved in it: (1) it's a club, and it belongs to its members; (2) all members are aware that their presence is expected and their absence will be missed—people need to be needed; (3) members must have opportunities to be together socially; (4) Fountain House cannot neglect the circumstances in which people live, so an apartment program is one of its goals (Beard, Propst, & Malamud, 1982).

As a result of the 1976 NIMH grant to provide training in the clubhouse model, seventy-seven programs began using Fountain House methods by 1980, and in 1981, the first international conference was hosted by a clubhouse in Pakistan (Mandiberg & Edwards, 2013). In 1987, another grant led to the development of the International Center for Clubhouse Development (ICCD), located on Tenth Avenue in New York. The ICCD, also referred to as Clubhouse International, maintains separate offices from Fountain House and has a six-fold mission: expansion, accreditation, training, research, advocacy, and public awareness (http://www.iccd.org/index.htmlex.html). At the fifth international seminar in 1989, the clubhouse community adopted a set of thirty-six standards to be used for clubhouse certification.

Mandiberg and Edwards (2013) have advanced the concept of collective identity formation within the clubhouse culture. Having a collective identity that is positive is more salient for the recovering individual than having a relational identity with a care provider (mental health professional); thus, the clubhouse culture becomes more powerful than a relationship, however positive, with a therapist. Furthermore, "the origins of the clubhouse model in mutual aid lead clubhouses to intentionally limit staff and define staff roles and skills as primarily facilitating and sharing work" (Mandiberg & Edwards, 2013, p. 27). In this way, the clubhouse is intrinsically different from other mental health settings. In addition, the clubhouse sponsors multiple activities that lead to friendship and mutual aid, where the "stigma, stereotyping, and exclusion" of the outside world are eliminated (p. 28). Weak ties with more people are more likely to buffer stigma and discrimination than strong dyadic relationships, a point reminiscent of Granovetter's "strength of weak ties" (Granovetter, 1973; Mandiberg & Edwards, 2013). Collective identity, like that found in the clubhouse, is inherently more strengthening than an identity created in dyadic relationships like those formed with psychotherapists.

Financing

Funding for Fountain House comes from multiple sources, mainly from private support in the form of foundation and organization grants but also from individual contributions, fundraising events, and investment income from an endowment. It also receives fees and grants from government agencies, program service fees, gallery art sales, training tuition, and other sources, for a total in 2012 of $17,294,228. As of 2012, Fountain House in New York served 1,300 members (https://www.fountainhouse.org/content/about/financials).

Diffusion

The Fountain House working community model has inspired more than four hundred clubhouses in thirty-two states and thirty countries. These programs serve more than 55,000 people with serious mental illness (http://www.idealist.org/view/org/cFZtphbS2ZMD).

Success Rates

The Fountain House website (https://www.fountainhouse.org/content/about) reports the following outcome figures:

1. Seventy-seven percent of participants in Fountain House's Education Program complete their studies. The average education completion rate for students with mental illness is thirty-two percent.
2. Sixty-five percent of Fountain House members have achieved employment through the employment program. The average employment rate for people with mental illness is fifteen percent.
3. Members receiving psychiatric services at the Sidney Baer Center, which integrates psychiatric and primary healthcare, have a relapse rate of seven percent. The current average relapse rate for similarly diagnosed individuals is fifty percent.

CONCLUSION

In his historical review of the impact of the US government on the mental health treatment system, E. F. Torrey (2014) lists existing state programs that could have been models for the community centers created by legislation for federal support of mental health but were not. He enumerates thirteen, in thirteen different states, but there are others. Among those listed were the Fairweather Lodge and Fountain

TABLE 12.1
COMPARISON OF FAIRWEATHER LODGES, OXFORD HOUSES, AND FOUNTAIN HOUSE

	Fairweather Lodges	Oxford Houses	Fountain House
Founding	1963, Palo Alto, California	1975, Silver Spring, Maryland	1948, New York City
Founder	George Fairweather	J. Paul Molloy	John Beard
Members	People with mental health conditions	Alcoholics/addicts	People with mental health conditions
Number of houses 2013	90 lodges in 16 states	1,612 houses in 45 states and 6 foreign countries, providing 12,735 beds	400+ clubhouses in 30 countries and 32 states.
Financing	Partially self-supporting with help from local governments and contributions	Houses are self-supporting; administration and recruitment funded by government, contributions, and grants	Foundation/ organization grants, contributions from individuals, fundraisers, fees and grants from government, services fees, training tuition
Annual budget	$10,631,345 for one program with 302 adults in multiple lodges (Minnesota)	A single house budget requires no funding other than member contributions	$17,294,228 for Fountain House in New York, with 1,300 members
Provides housing, employment, mutual support	Yes, all three, except that many residents are on social security disability rather than working	Yes, housing and mutual support; helps with independent employment	Yes, mutual support for all members, housing for those who need it, employment for those who want it

House, both of which rely on mutual support among members and on few professional staffers. Both programs had been established before the Community Mental Health Centers legislation in 1965 and had proven cost-effective. The National Institute of Mental Health has awarded funds to both. This is but one of the many unfathomable oversights by mental health policy makers in the last half-century.

Toward the end of his analysis, Torrey says of Fountain House: "In addition to medication, individuals with serious mental illnesses need access to decent housing, vocational opportunities, and opportunities for socialization. The clubhouse model is the best model for meetings those needs" (Torrey, 2014, p. 155).

Two points in this chapter bear special notice. One is how similar Fairweather's experience in trying to disseminate his program was to Low's efforts to get hospitals to adopt will-training groups in state hospitals twenty-two years earlier. Another is how difficult it has been to implement community mental health innovations, compared with how relatively swiftly the Oxford Houses caught on. I say relatively because it took the Anti-Drug Abuse Act of 1988 and the amendments to the Federal Fair Housing Act in the same year to facilitate the development of Oxford Houses thirteen years after they began in 1975. And, as Molloy pointed out in his 2012 interview with Bill White, Oxford Houses serve a small percentage of the alcoholics and addicts in treatment in any given year, and those in treatment represent only one in ten of those who are addicted. A point in favor of Oxford Houses' development is their relationship with the self-help communities of AA and NA. These fellowships, with their extensive networks, support house members' integration back into community life and help sustain the houses as independent entities in the community. Table 12.1 compares the three programs.

The next, and last, chapter covers online groups and the various ways those seeking help can access and use them.

REFERENCES

Anderson, S. B. (1998). *Fountain House and the development of clubhouse culture*. New York, NY: Fountain House.

Beard, J. H., Propst, R. N., & Malamud, T. J. (1982). The Fountain House model of psychiatric rehabilitation. *Psychosocial Rehabilitation Journal, 5*(1), 1–13.

Doyle, A., Lanoil, J., & Dudek, K. (2013). *Fountain House: Creating community in mental health practice*. New York, NY: Columbia University Press.

Fairweather, G. W. (1980). Spreading the lodge society concept. In G. E. Fairweather (Ed.), *The Fairweather Lodge: A twenty-five year retrospective* (pp. 33–42). San Francisco, CA: Jossey-Bass.

Fairweather, G. W. (1994). *Keeping the balance: A psychologist's story*. Austin, TX: Fairweather Publishing.

Fairweather, G. W., Sanders, D. H., Maynard, H., & Cressler, D. L. (with Bleck, D. S.). (1969). *Community life for the mentally ill: An alternative to institutional care*. Chicago, IL: Aldine.

Fergus, E. (1980). Maintaining and advancing the lodge effort. In G. E. Fairweather (Ed.), *The Fairweather Lodge: A twenty-five year retrospective* (pp. 43–56). San Francisco, CA: Jossey Bass.

Granovetter, M. (1973). The strength of weak ties. *American Journal of Sociology, 78*, 1360–1380.

Jason, L. A., Olson, B. D., & Foli, K. (2008). *Rescued lives: The Oxford House approach to substance abuse*. New York, NY: Routledge.

Low, A. (1943/1991). *Mental illness, stigma and self-help*. Glencoe, IL: Willet Publishing.

Mandiberg, J. M., & Edwards, M. (2013). Collective identity formation in the mental health clubhouse community. *International Journal of Self-Help and Self-Care*, *7*(1), 19–39.

Mateer, W. (1980). The lodge as a private non-profit corporation. In G. E. Fairweather (Ed.), *The Fairweather Lodge: A twenty-five year retrospective* (pp. 81–86). San Francisco, CA: Jossey-Bass.

Oxford House. (2011.) *Oxford House manual*. Available at http://www.oxfordhouse.org/userfiles/file/doc/man_house.pdf

Oxford House. (2012). Annual report. *Oxford House good neighbors—good citizens*. Available at http://www.oxfordhouse.org/userfiles/file/doc/ar2011.pdf

Rapp, C. A., & Goscha, R. J. (2012). *The strengths model: A recovery-oriented approach to mental health services* (3rd ed.). New York, NY: Oxford University Press.

Torrey, E. F. (2014). *American psychosis: How the federal government destroyed the mental illness treatment system*. New York, NY: Oxford University Press.

White, W. L. (2012). The Oxford House story: An interview with Paul Molloy. www.williamwhitepapers.com/leadership_interviews/recovery_management_interviews

Existing research survey data, combined with anecdotal observations and case reports, indicate that members of online self-help groups receive benefits that go beyond what face-to-face (f2f) groups can offer.

KING & MOREGGI (2007, p. 240)

13

ONLINE GROUPS

ONLINE SUPPORT GROUPS are popular with consumers; 28 percent of a self-selected sample of online users in the United States indicated that their online searches are mostly for online support groups (Ybarra & Eaton 2005). Most support and self-help mutual-aid groups maintain a presence online by way of the Internet and on the World Wide Web. This online presence is of two basic kinds: sites offering information and sites making possible participation.

Most of the informational sites are websites that allow those interested (1) to learn more about the group, (2) to learn the locations of actual in-person meetings if the group offers them, and (3) to learn how to contact by e-mail or telephone some source of further information. Those who know of the existence of a specific group should have no difficulty accessing its online presence. The websites of many such groups also serve members, offering literature and suggestions for helpful readings. A good example is the site of Narcotics Anonymous (http://www.na.org). On this site, one finds information about NA from its biennial surveys, access to publication ordering, information on NA's service projects, discussion boards, and much more.

Table 13.1 shows the subtypes of online support groups. These types are not mutually exclusive; for example, a group might be both nonprofessionally hosted and online-only. Support groups, such as Psychobabble, hosted by a professional (Hsiung, 2000) are probably the least available. Some online participation sites of each kind are synchronous, offering real-time meetings and/or chat rooms, such as Marijuana Anonymous (http://www.ma-online.org/chat.php), while others are asynchronous, making available forums or opportunities for e-mail exchanges. Many participation sites offer both. Most allow both members and nonmembers to "lurk," or observe at least some activity on the site without participating or even revealing their presence.

TABLE 13.1
TYPES OF ONLINE GROUPS

Type	Example
Face-to-face with an online component	Moderation Management (http://www.moderation.org)
Online-only	Bipolar Significant Others (http://www.bpso.org)
Synchronous (i.e., chat and real-time)	Marijuana Anonymous (http://www.ma-online.org/chat.php)
Asynchronous (i.e., e-mail forums)	Mental Health Forum (http://www.mentalhealthforum.net)
Professionally hosted	Psychobabble (http://www.dr-bob.org/babble/social)
Nonprofessionally hosted	Recovery International Online (http://www.lowselfhelpsystems.org/meetings/online-meetings.asp

Participation practices for online meetings and chat rooms differ. Most sites offer clear instructions, and people needing more guidance will almost always be offered help, especially after identifying themselves as "newbies." Somewhat different from forums and chat rooms are newsgroups or listservs, a kind of group e-mail in which each message that is posted goes to all group members, who receive it either individually as it is sent or in a kind of summary digest at the end of each day. Listservs are often moderated: each message passes through a group monitor who has responsibility for ensuring that it is relevant to the concerns of the group and does not violate group standards of proper language and so on. Listservs and other asynchronous modes seem to offer a special advantage. The therapeutic value of writing about one's thoughts and feelings may alleviate depression and loneliness and reduce pain and stress (Smyth, Stone, Hurewitz, & Kaell, 1999). Several studies of online groups have reported that members feel a sense of catharsis after sending messages to their groups (Miller & Gergen, 1998; Finn, 1999; White & Dorman, 2000). In this respect, online groups have a distinct advantage over traditional groups, where participation may not give a person enough time to think through what he or she says.

Information about and links to all these kinds of groups may be found in box 13.1. There are many other sites, as searches for "support groups" or "self-help groups" will attest. Despite their label, however, many of these groups have a professional or profit-making connection.

BOX 13.1
GUIDES TO ONLINE RESOURCES

John Grohol's Psych Central (http://psychcentral.com/resources)
National Mental Health Consumers' Self-Help Clearinghouse (http://www.mhself-help.org)
American Self-Help Clearinghouse Sourcebook Online (http://www.mentalhelp.net/selfhelp)
Faces & Voices of Recovery Guide to Mutual Aid Resources (http://www.facesandvoicesofrecovery.org/resources/support/resources/online.html11

Although some plateaus have apparently been reached in the "wiring" of the United States and Canada, the continuing proliferation of mobile devices such as tablets and smartphones and the likelihood of continuing increases in bandwidth suggest that the number of Web users will continue to grow. Full participation in all groups may not always be available to all individuals, but with the availability of free e-mail programs that allow private storage on the Web itself, even someone who must rely on a public library terminal can participate in the many available e-mail-based groups (DeAndrea & Anthony, 2013).

But there is need for caution as we approach this topic; the study of peer-support groups requires respect. As Barak, Grohol, and Pector (2004, p. 1166) cautioned, "research of online peer-to-peer support groups by professionals is rather paternalistic, and it completely misses the point that the Internet environment is viewed by its users as a self-empowering medium. Users do not necessarily want, or need, professional researchers present in peer-to-peer support groups, which are run by ordinary people for ordinary people."

UTILITY AND BENEFITS OF ONLINE GROUPS AND MEETINGS

When and why might online participation in a support or self-help mutual-aid group be beneficial, useful, or even necessary? One notable advantage of Web-based groups is their ability to reach special populations. Computer contact reduces barriers of time, distance, and social status, allowing persons with physical disabilities, home-bound caregivers, status-conscious professionals, and individuals in remote locations the opportunity to participate actively and on an equal basis with the more advantaged (Cudney & Weinert, 2000; Perron, 2002; Weinert, Cudney, & Winters, 2005). Beder (2005) offers a vivid and detailed description of the importance of a variety of online resources to a professional social worker who had to become a caregiver.

Shy adolescents, many of whom have not sought professional treatment and some who have sought treatment but not made substantial changes during primary treatment, have made significant breakthroughs online (Humphreys & Klaw, 2001). Those who view themselves as stigmatized are especially attracted to online resources (Cooper, 2004). As Salem, Bogat, and Reid noted as early as 1997 (p. 189): "On-line mutual help may provide a unique form of support for persons who are not as likely to use traditional forms of helping." Also, of course, "computer-mediated social support groups may provide people with a network of individuals to whom they can turn for support when needs are not being met by traditional providers of support" (Wright & Bell, 2003, p. 49).

A case in point is the canine epilepsy group to which I belong. This is an e-mail listserv moderated and assisted by a select group of members who have special knowledge of the subject in addition to personal experience. It is their role to screen for possible listserv members from among those who initially approach the website for information about canine epilepsy. Each list member has been offered a place on the listserv following an exchange of information about the dog and its illness. There is no other avenue to membership on the list.

Although this is not a mental health site, its members qualify as stressed, at times extremely so. Canine epilepsy can be difficult to treat. Dogs with the illness are triggered by a wide variety of toxic substances and allergies, or alternatively, there may be no rhyme or reason to the dog's seizures. Some dogs will respond well to an antiseizure drug and stabilize right away; others seem refractory to almost any combination of various expensive drugs. Members remain on the list as long as they feel they need it. Once a dog's illness is stabilized, many members reduce participation but still remain in contact in order to offer support to other members when crises erupt. In addition, when dogs become ill with conditions other than epilepsy, members are free to ask for help in the form of experiential knowledge and support.

Some owners of epileptic dogs become extremely sensitized to their pets if the dogs' seizures are not controlled. Never knowing when the dog is going to suddenly go into a grand-mal seizure makes the owner jumpy and protective; this is an example of how just about any support group could be seen as a mental health resource. The epilepsy listserv includes members from all over the world, which is one of the advantages of online participation. There are not enough of us to establish a local group, and we probably would not attend a face-to-face group anyway. Most of the members can get support from others online at any time of the day or night, where otherwise the individual would be left at home waiting until the veterinary office opened the next morning.

Early in the computer age, males far outnumbered female users. But this changed rapidly in the twenty-first century, when a high percentage of women began to utilize online support groups, a phenomenon attributable to the groups' accessibility, convenience, and safety, along with their ability to provide gender-based services in a stigma-free format to women in communities that lack local women's recovery support group meetings. Hall and Tidwell's (2003) study of those using Internet-based recovery-support services reported that women made up more than 60 percent of those using such services, a dramatically higher percentage than that found in treatment admissions and surveys of face-to-face recovery-support groups.

Others for whom this format could offer special advantages include status-conscious professionals (e.g., physicians, business executives, judges), adolescents (Skinner, Maley, Smith, Chirrey, & Morrison, 2001), persons with impairments that limit access to or usefulness of face-to-face meetings (e.g., persons with hearing loss) (Cummings, Sproull, & Kiesler, 2002), individuals in remote locations (e.g., those living in rural or reservation communities), and those who have not sought professional treatment, including nondependent drinkers (Humphreys & Klaw, 2001). What Salem et al. noted in 1997 (p. 189) has changed somewhat but far from totally:

> In spite of the growing popularity [of self-help and support groups], there are impediments to participation. First, in sparsely populated areas, it may be difficult to find a sufficient number of persons who share the same problem, and, even if sufficient numbers are found to begin a group, attending meetings may involve considerable travel time and expense (Adam & Hoehne, 1989; Madara, 1992). Second, many individuals feel uncomfortable disclosing personal information in a face-to-face setting because of concerns regarding confidentiality, anonymity, and stigmatization (Levy & Derby, 1992).

Many groups are not conveniently located or may meet at times or on days that render attendance difficult for some. There are also the home-bound. In a rapidly aging society, for one example, some caregivers may find in-person meeting attendance difficult or even at times impossible (Colvin, Chenoweth, Bold, & Harding, 2004; Powell, Chiu, & Eysenbach, 2008). And it is likely precisely at such times that the caregiver may really experience "needing a meeting." This is also where a harried caregiver will likely find others in the same or similar situations, enabling a special experience of healing identification.

Another situation inviting online participation is that of the ill member or one recovering at home after surgery or some other circumstance that limits mobility. Some groups make heroic efforts to "bring the meeting" to someone thus handicapped, but this is not always possible. There are also situations in which a member may for one reason or another become dissatisfied with the available in-person meeting choices. One example would be the militantly agnostic or atheistic AA member who finds objectionable the prayer practice of an otherwise available meeting.

KINDS OF PARTICIPATION

Online participation takes several forms. There are actual meetings with a variety of participants, some with the possibility of visual contact afforded by Skype—for example, many NA meetings. There are also synchronous meetings and chat rooms, where participants engage in actual real-time dialogue and exchanges. The most ready example of these may be found in the many AA meetings listed at http://aa-intergroup.org/directory.php. The same site lists asynchronous meetings that use forums or e-mail. These offer time for more thought between postings, which can be either advantageous or the opposite.

Lurkers are a separate but important category. Most who read this book will probably at least begin their online explorations in this way. But so will many who are interested in but perhaps ambivalent about taking part in a group. Most who join any group after its start-up probably observe—or lurk—before committing to membership. Although many view lurkers as freeloaders who seek to gain without contributing, most serious research on the phenomenon suggests that this is a poor understanding. Nonnecke and Preece (1999, 2000, 2001, 2003) and Preece, Nonnecke, and Andrews (2004), who have most intensively researched lurking, urge that it be seen as a behavior reflecting the users' needs and reasons, and these can be personal (entertainment, curiosity, and learning), to satisfy information needs, to learn about the group, to maintain privacy and safety, to reduce noise and exposure on the site, to act within constraints, and to act in response to group dynamics.

One reason the majority of lurkers choose not to post is that they are reading and browsing, and that may be enough for them. All users need to read before they can engage in any other activity. Lurkers are active; they are reading rather than ignoring the material. In a sense, all users are at some point lurkers, reading before engaging in another activity. Lurking can also be understood as listening, lurkers serving as a conventional mass-media audience (Edelmann, 2013). Some online groups encourage lurking because it helps new users get a feeling for the group, the kind of people who participate in it, and how it operates. At the same time, lurkers may learn vicariously by reading about the experiences that other participants report (van Uden-Kraan, Drossaert, Taal, Seydel, & van de Laar, 2008).

POSITIVE VALUES

Despite some concerns that we will examine in the next section, research suggests that participation in online groups benefits people in many ways. First and most obviously, it allows the curious to get some idea of just what a group is all about. As King and Moreggi (1998, p. 85) noted, "some people have their first contact with self-help organizations by their online presence. There are documented cases of drug addicts who became willing to give up a destructive habit for the first time after witnessing the conversations between members of a recovery online self-help group." It is also true that online groups develop their own sense of community, often as strong as that experienced through actual physical presence (Eysenbach, Powell, Englesakis, Rizo, & Stern, 2004).

Existing research survey data, combined with anecdotal observations and case reports, in fact suggest that members of online self-help groups receive benefits that go beyond what face-to-face groups can offer (Lamberg 2003). Perhaps because of the anonymity afforded online, a higher level of self-disclosure seems to take place in these groups. Research indicates that people self-disclose a greater degree of sensitive information online than they do in person (Newman, Consoli, & Barr, 1997). For a particular example, Pistrang, Barker, and Humphreys (2008, p. 117) noted that in "the only study of internet support groups, Houston, Cooper & Ford (2002) used a longitudinal design to assess depressive symptoms over time. One-third of members showed a resolution of depressive symptoms with more frequent users more likely to improve (after adjusting for a number of other variables)." The investigators had been concerned that use of an online support group might have the unfortunate consequence of decreasing face-to-face social support, but they found that social support scores did not change over time.

Salem et al. (1997, p. 202) found that "online groups have unique characteristics that distinguish them from their face-to-face counterparts—higher levels of expressed emotional support and self-disclosure, less formal structure and group process, and greater participation by men."

DISADVANTAGES AND CONCERNS

There have been concerns from the beginning about possible problems springing from the use of online groups. Does participation in online groups make it more likely or less likely that such participants will also join in-person, face-to-face groups? One worry over the years has been that the availability of online participation in a group might inhibit some individuals from seeking actual face-to-face contact; they would "bury themselves in their computers" (Goldberger, 1995). Caplan (2003,

p. 626) suggested that "problematic psychosocial predispositions lead individuals to excessive and compulsive computer-mediated social interaction, which, in turn, worsens their problems." A reflection of this concern may be found in a December 2005 posting to the NA "Online Recovery" site, reposted in January 2007.

> We strongly urge people to consider carefully what they are doing before they share *anonymously* online and to know that things and people are not always what they may seem to be and most often are not. Please get involved in real life recovery at NA meetings in your area. Please, turn off your computers and get involved in real life in your recovery and in your community today. Life can be worth living if you go for it.

Although NA is more resistant than other groups, it is not unique in its concern that online presence and interaction are not as healing for some individuals as are regular face-to-face encounters. Openness to online participation developed slowly. As Madara noted in 1997 (p. 23), it had been the "maverick members of some national and international self-help groups [who] were the first to establish online self-help meetings." Mavericks are not usually followed. Thus, it is not surprising that, as Madara went on to note, "it has only been within the last two years that most self-help group headquarters have finally developed their own online presence."

A related source of concern was early research finding that those who participated in peer-to-peer support group programs reported on "the Internet paradox": a decrease in satisfaction with the emotional support they received from preexisting relationships (Kraut et al., 1998) and an increase in negative interactions with the members of their original support network (Helgeson, Cohen, Schulz, & Yasko, 1999). Those who join an online support group and build close relationships therein can develop highly idealized perceptions of other users (Wright & Bell, 2003), which can result in a preference for social interaction in online groups over offline interaction in face-to-face settings (Chung, 2013).

Later research by the same scholars shed a different light on this concern. Kraut et al. (2002, p. 49) reported that a "3-year follow-up of 208 of these respondents found that negative effects dissipated." While conceding that "maturation of [the] participants" may explain part of this change, the researchers determined that "a change in the nature of the Internet is the most parsimonious explanation ... the Internet provided a richer supply of information, with more news, health, financial, hobby, work, community, and consumer information available" (pp. 68–69). For members of self-help and support groups, it seems a fair inference that the increasing online availability of those groups was part of the "richer supply" that allowed for greater appreciation of offline interactions.

A final occasional difficulty is that inaccurate and outdated information can spread, because online groups do not necessarily limit who can author and post (Coulson, 2005); however, research has shown that most incorrect and unreliable information is corrected by other members fairly soon after it is posted (Chung, 2013, citing Esquivel, Meric-Bernstam, & Bernstam, 2006).

AREAS OF UNCERTAINTY OR CONCERN

Online groups differ from their face-to-face counterparts in several ways. First and most obviously, online contact affords a different type of privacy and anonymity. Except for some users of Skype, there is no visual contact. First names, when used, may offer a hint about gender, but such visually obvious traits as race, disability, and age are masked. This is a different kind of privacy and anonymity, a very real kind of invisibility. This may be related to one gender difference that researchers have noted in support group postings: men are twice as likely to give or ask for information related to a disorder, while women use the group to share personal experiences and provide encouragement and support (White & Dorman, 2001; Klemm, Hurst, Dearholt, & Trone, 1999).

Ensured invisibility raises another concern: the disinhibition that online communication fosters (Kiesler, Siegel, & McGuire, 1984; Sproull & Kiesler, 1984). As one investigator summarized: "If all computer-mediated communication systems can be said to have one single unifying effect upon human behavior, it is that usage tends to cause the user to become less inhibited" (Reid, 1994, p. 19). Many have seen this as an advantage. Griffiths (2005, p. 556), for example, suggested that freedom from pressures for social desirability "may lead to increased levels of honesty and, therefore, higher validity in the case of self-disclosure. The Internet may, as a consequence, provide access to socially unskilled individuals who may not have sought help if it were not for the online nature of the self-help group."

But the impact of this disinhibition effect on an online support group can be both negative and positive (Barak, Boniel-Nissim, & Suler, 2008; Tanis, 2007; Tanis & Postmes, 2007). Because honesty and self-disclosure are such important therapeutic ingredients of these groups, the disinhibition effect can accelerate salutary functions. Group members might reveal secret emotions, fears, or wishes; they might show unusual kindness. As a result, interpersonal intimacy and group bonding develop. However, the disinhibition effect may not always be so benign. It can also lead to rude language, harsh criticism, anger, hatred, and even threats. For others, self-disclosure might develop too rapidly, resulting in regret, anxiety, and a hasty termination of membership in the group.

Insofar as self-disclosure lies at the heart of all self-help and support group processes, the reciprocity of self-disclosure that characterizes online groups helps to render them especially effective (Barak & Gluck-Ofri, 2007). The protection given by anonymity opens new possibilities to explore roles and styles. As the famous *New Yorker* cartoon put it, "On the Internet nobody knows you're a dog" (July 5, 1993, p. 61). Especially in asynchronous settings—when there is a time lapse between communications—the self may be crafted in ways that transmit fuller truths. But disinhibition may twist self-disclosure; imaginations may on occasion run wild.

One danger in this possibility is what psychiatrist Marc Feldman (2000, p. 669) has labeled "Munchausen by Internet," the online propagation of factitious illness or crisis: "individuals willfully feign or induce illness in themselves or in others.... Their goal is emotional gratification from taking the sick role. Instead of seeking care at numerous hospitals, these individuals can now gain new audiences merely by clicking from one support group to another." The obvious problem with such usage is not so much "wasted empathy" as the tendency of such experiences to breed mistrust and so to impede the identification that undergirds much of the healing that takes place in self-help and support groups (Caspi & Gorsky, 2006; Pulman & Taylor, 2011).

THE DANGER OF EXPLOITATION

As some have noted, the World Wide Web can at times become a new Wicked Wild West; various con and scam artists populate the Web as they do just about all other social spaces. While the groups listed on the Grohol and the Faces & Voices of Recovery websites (see box 13.1) are generally trustworthy, the Web as a whole is only slightly less chaotic—and may be more than slightly more dangerous—than wandering through the dark alleys of a neighborhood that the area's residents avoid. Those Web-worldly-wise know how to recognize and avoid such traps, but even some who think themselves sophisticated in this area have on occasion stumbled. Three areas merit special concern: privacy, finances, and sexuality.

In the case of privacy, the very nature of self-help mutual-aid and support groups is such that a degree of intimacy is a regular part of their process. Self-disclosure begets self-disclosure, and the atmosphere of mutual trust over shared vulnerability tends to elicit a type of honesty not found in most other settings. Privacy involves control over what is known about oneself. The Internet, it is good to remember, is like a postcard: it may be addressed to one individual or small group, but it is at least possible and may even be likely that it can be read wantonly by many others.

With regard to finances, as self-help guru Ed Madara pointed out years ago, "Once professionals see the parade, they run to the front to lead it" (personal communication, 3-29-07) Many who offer professional services online are legitimate; many others are not. A fair number of the goods and services offered are of a somewhat shoddy or at least dubious nature. But there may also be a deeper psychological danger. Not all who offer help are competent to do so. And in the areas of both mental health and addiction services, the very nature of the problem of those seeking help often leads them to seek out and prefer easy answers and simple solutions. One important responsibility of those devoted to genuine recovery must be to guard and, if possible, guide those help seekers who because of their very disability are vulnerable to the maneuvers of those less interested in serving them than in exploiting them.

Most well-formed self-help mutual-aid and support groups know of professionals whom members can trust. This may be most obvious in matters medical and financial, but it can extend to a very specific version of an "Angie's List." Those in the midst of suffering tend to be more vulnerable; already in some sense wounded, they both wound more easily and can more easily be manipulated by those promising to heal them. One role of a helping paraprofessional in such settings may be the quiet, careful overseeing of the kinds of referrals members offer one another. This can extend to suggestions about care in using Web resources.

Although appeals for money are in general to be distrusted, a few online groups request donations. One example is the online intergroup of AA, which follows the seventh tradition of self-support, just as face-to-face AA groups do. In these cases, the "donation" is genuinely such, totally optional; giving does not bring special status, privilege, or advantage.

The third prevalent danger is sexual. Those who are in some way disabled can be especially vulnerable to those who explicitly or implicitly seem to promise caring. There is a special loneliness in disability, in being set off from others because of some kind of deficiency or difference. This is one reason self-help mutual-aid groups have such healing power: they make whole in the context of "shared honesty [about] mutual vulnerability" (Kurtz, 1979, p. 61). This is another area in which well-formed groups, online or face-to-face, quietly but watchfully protect newcomers. Some online groups encourage sponsorship, a special relationship between a kind of mentor and someone striving for growth. Except for sponsor relationships, however, veteran members discourage dyadic pairing off. A group is a group.

Some helpful articles on these aspects of online support groups may be found online at http://www.selfhelpmagazine.com/search/node/online%20 groups. Especially useful may be the lead article, "The Secret to Staying Safe in Online Support Groups" (http://www.selfhelpmagazine.com/articles/online-support-groups). Forums are also offered at http://selfhelpmagazine.com/forum, although most are not kept as up-to-date as the forums on the websites of particular groups.

CONCLUSION

Once upon a time, when families were larger and more extended, when neighborhoods were more stable and just about everyone belonged to an active parish church or synagogue that sponsored various kinds of associations, when intergenerational mobility was measured more in steps than by leaps, the idea of self-help mutual-aid and support groups would have seemed both far-fetched and obvious. "But that's what we do!" many would have exclaimed, hearing their description, even as others slowly shook their heads in puzzlement and wondered, "But why would people do that?"

The expansion of the word "community" by the adjective "online" has created similar bemusement. The small-group revolution that began in the 1930s with AA and Recovery, Inc., at the end of the twentieth century produced its own unanticipated generation of offspring. How would a subculture in which hugging was common currency adapt to connection by esoteric symbols? Could those who ridiculed "Ma Bell's" urging to "Reach out and touch someone" find healing in relationships in which even the voice was absent?

So far, for some, the answer seems affirmative. But just as self-help and support groups themselves are not for everyone, their online variations require more than technical adeptness in those who would use them for human contact. The healing that takes place when injury meets injury cannot be commanded, face-to-face or online. Online self-help and support groups, like their in-person parents, can usefully be tried, approached with curious open-mindedness. But here as elsewhere in the reality of human life, there is no one, best, final way that will suit all. Human beings differ, and so, therefore, must the modalities that serve them. The realities of twenty-first-century communication offer rich new modalities, but their proof must be in their results. There is no one best way for everyone, in anything.

REFERENCES

Adam, D., & Hoehne, D. (1989). Mutual aid in remote areas: Addressing the obstacles. *Canada's Mental Health, 37*, 18–21.

Barak, A., Boniel-Nissim, M., & Suler, J. (2008). Fostering empowerment in online support groups. *Computers in Human Behavior, 24*(5), 1867–1883.

Barak, A., & Gluck-Ofri, O. (2007). Degree and reciprocity of self-disclosure in online forums. *Cyberpsychology and Behavior, 10*(3), 407–417.

Barak, A., Grohol, J. M., & Pector, E. (2004). Methodology, validity, and applicability: A critique on Eysenbach et al. *British Medical Journal, 328*, 1166.

Beder, J. (2005). Cybersolace: Technology built on emotion. *Social Work, 50*(4), 355–358.

Caplan, S. E. (2003). Preference for online social interaction: A theory of problematic Internet use and psychosocial well-being. *Communication Research, 30*, 625–648.

Caspi, A., & Gorsky, P. (2006). Online deception: Prevalence, motivation, and emotion. *Cyberpsychology and Behavior, 9*(1), 54–59.

Chung, J. E. (2013). Social interaction in online support groups: Preference for online social interaction over offline social interaction. *Computers in Human Behavior, 29*(4), 1408–1414.

Colvin, J., Chenoweth, L., Bold, M., & Harding, C. (2004). Caregivers of older adults: Advantages and disadvantages of Internet-based social support. *Family Relations, 53*(1), 49–57.

Cooper, G. (2004). Exploring and understanding online assistance for problem gamblers: The pathways disclosure model. *International Journal of Mental Health and Addiction, 1*(2), 32–38.

Coulson, N. S. (2005). Receiving social support online: An analysis of a computer-mediated support group for individuals living with irritable bowel syndrome. *Cyberpsychology and Behavior, 8*(6), 580–584.

Cudney, S. A., & Weinert, C. (2000). Computer-based support groups: Nursing in cyberspace. *Computers in Nursing, 18*(1), 35–43.

Cummings, J. N., Sproull, L., & Kiesler, S. B. (2002). Beyond hearing: Where real-world and online support meet. *Group Dynamics, 6*(1), 78–88.

DeAndrea, D. C., & Anthony, J. C. (2013). Online peer support for mental health problems in the United States: 2004–2010. *Psychological Medicine, 43*(11), 2277–2288.

Edelmann, N. (2013). Reviewing the definitions of "lurkers" and some implications for online research. *Cyberpsychology, Behavior, and Social Networking, 16*(9), 645–649.

Esquivel, A., Meric-Bernstam, F., & Bernstam, E. V. (2006). Accuracy and self correction of information received from an Internet breast cancer list: Content analysis. *British Medical Journal, 332*(7547), 939–942.

Eysenbach, G., Powell, J., Englesakis, M., Rizo, C., & Stern, A. (2004). Health related virtual communities and electronic support groups: Systematic review of the effects of online peer to peer interactions. *British Medical Journal, 328*(7449), 1166.

Feldman, M. D. (2000). Munchausen by Internet: Detecting factitious illness and crisis on the Internet. *Southern Medical Journal, 93*(7), 669–672.

Finn, J. (1999). An exploration of helping processes in an online self-help group focusing on issues of disability. *Health and Social Work, 24*(3), 220–231.

Goldberger, P. (1995, October 5). Cyberspace trips to nowhere land. *New York Times*. http://www.nytimes.com/1995/10/05/garden/design-notebook-cyberspace-trips-to-nowhere-land.html?src=pm&pagewanted=2

Griffiths, M. (2005). Online therapy for addictive behaviors. *Cyberpsychology and Behavior, 8*(6), 555–561.

Hall, M. J., & Tidwell, W. C. (2003). Internet recovery for substance abuse and alcoholism: An exploratory study of service users. *Journal of Substance Abuse Treatment, 24*(2), 161–167.

Helgeson, V. S., Cohen, S., Schulz, R., & Yasko, J. (1999). Education and peer discussion group interventions and adjustment to breast cancer. *Archives of General Psychiatry, 56*(4), 340.

Houston, T. K., Cooper, L. A., & Ford, D. (2002). Internet support groups for depression: A 1-year prospective cohort study. *American Journal of Psychiatry, 159*,
Hsiung, R. C. (2000). The best of both worlds: An online self-help group hosted by a mental health professional. *Cyberpsychology and Behavior, 3*(6), 935–950.
Humphreys, K., & Klaw, E. (2001). Can targeting nondependent problem drinkers and providing Internet-based services expand access to assistance for alcohol problems? A study of the moderation management self-help/mutual aid organization. *Journal of Studies on Alcohol, 62*(4), 528–532.
Kiesler, S., Siegel, J., & McGuire, T. W. (1984). Social psychological aspects of computer-mediated communication. *American Psychologist, 39*(10), 1123–1134.
King, S. A., & Moreggi, D. (1998). Internet self-help and support groups: The pros and cons. In J. Gackenback (Ed.), *Psychology and the Internet: Intrapersonal, interpersonal and transpersonal implications* (pp. 77–109). San Diego, CA: Academic Press.
King, S. A., & Moreggi, D. (2006). Internet self-help and support groups: The pros and cons of text-based mutual aid. In J. Gackenbach (Ed.), *Psychology and the Internet: Intrapersonal, interpersonal and transpersonal implications* 2nd ed. (pp. 221–244). San Diego, CA: Academic Press.
Klemm, P., Hurst, M., Dearholt, S. L., & Trone, S. R. (1999). Cyber solace: Gender differences on Internet cancer support groups. *Computers in Nursing, 17*, 65–72.
Kraut, R. E., Patterson, M., Lundmark, V., Kiesler, S., Mukhopadhyay, T., & Scherlis, W. (1998). Internet paradox: A social technology that reduces social involvement and psychological well-being? *American Psychologist, 53*(9), 1017–1032.
Kraut, R., Kiesler, S., Boneva, B., Cummings, J., Helgeson, V., & Crawford, A. (2002). Internet paradox revisited. *Journal of Social Issues, 58*(1), 49–74.
Kurtz, E. (1979). *Not-God: A history of Alcoholics Anonymous*. Center City, MN: Hazelden.
Lamberg, L. (2003). Online empathy for mood disorders. *JAMA, 289*(23), 3073–3077.
Levy, L. H., & Derby, J. F. (1992). Bereavement support groups: Who joins; who does not; and why. *American Journal of Community Psychology, 20*, 649–662.
Madara, E. (1992). The primary value of a self-help clearinghouse. In A. H. Katz, H. I. Hedrick, D. H. Isenberg, L. M. Thompson, T. Goodrich, & A. H. Kutscher (Eds.), *Self-help: Concepts and applications* (pp. 117–124). Philadelphia, PA: Charles Press.
Madara, E. (1997). The mutual-aid self-help online revolution. *Social Policy, 27*(3), 20–26.
Miller, J. K., & Gergen, K. J. (1998). Life on the line: The therapeutic potentials of computer mediated conversation. *Journal of Marital and Family Therapy, 24*(2), 189–202.
Newman, M. G., Consoli, A., & Barr, T. C. (1997). Computers in assessment and cognitive behavioral treatment of clinical disorders: Anxiety as a case in point. *Behavior Therapy, 28*, 211–235.
Nonnecke, B., & Preece, J. (1999). Shedding light on lurkers in online communities. In K. Buckner (Ed.), *Ethnographic studies in real and virtual environments: Inhabited information spaces and connected communities* (pp. 123–128). Edinburgh: Queen Margaret College.
Nonnecke, B., & Preece, J. (2000). Lurker demographics: Counting the silent. In *Proceedings of the SIGCHI Conference on Human Factors in Computing Systems* (pp. 73–80). The Hague, Netherlands. ACM. Available at http://www.acm.org/publications
Nonnecke, B., & Preece, J. (2001). Why lurkers lurk. In *Americas Conference on Information Systems* (pp. 1–10). Boston, MA. Available at http://aisel.aisnet.org/amcis2001

Nonnecke, B., & Preece, J. (2003). Silent participants: Getting to know lurkers better. In C. Lueg and D. Fisher (Eds.), *Usenet to CoWebs* (pp. 110–132). London: Springer.

Perron, B. (2002). Online support for caregivers of people with a mental illness. *Psychiatric Rehabilitation Journal, 26*(1), 70–77.

Pistrang, N., Barker, C., & Humphreys, K. (2008). Mutual help groups for mental health problems: A review of effectiveness studies. *American Journal of Community Psychology, 42*(1–2), 110–121.

Powell, J., Chiu, T., & Eysenbach, G. (2008). A systematic review of networked technologies supporting carers of people with dementia. *Journal of Telemedicine and Telecare, 14*(3), 154–156.

Preece, J., Nonnecke, B., & Andrews, D. (2004). The top five reasons for lurking: Improving community experiences for everyone. *Computers in Human Behavior, 20*(2), 201–223.

Pulman, A., & Taylor, J. (2012). Munchausen by Internet (MBI): Current research and future directions. *Journal of Medical Internet Research, 14*(4), 15.

Reid, E. M. (1994). *Cultural formations in text-based virtual realities* (Unpublished master's thesis). University of Melbourne, Australia. Available at http://www.aluluei.com/cult-form.htm

Salem, D. A., Bogat, G. A., & Reid, C. (1997). Mutual help goes online. *Journal of Community Psychology, 25*(2), 189–207.

Skinner, H., Maley, O., Smith, L., Chirrey, S., & Morrison, M. (2001). New frontiers: Using the Internet to engage teens in substance abuse prevention and treatment. In P. M. Monti, S. M. Colby, & T. A. O'Leary (Eds.), *Adolescents, alcohol, and substance abuse: Reaching teens through brief interventions* (pp. 297–318). New York, NY: Guilford.

Smyth, J. M., Stone, A. A., Hurewitz, A., & Kaell, A. (1999). Effects of writing about stressful experiences on symptom reduction in patients with asthma or rheumatoid arthritis. *JAMA, 281*(14), 1304–1309.

Sproull, L., & Kiesler, S. (1984). Encountering an alien culture. *Journal of Social Issues, 40*(3), 31–48.

Tanis, M. (2007). Online social support groups. In A. Joinson, K. Y. A. McKenna, T. Postmes, & U. D. Reips (Eds.), *Oxford handbook of Internet psychology* (pp. 137–152). Oxford: Oxford University Press.

Tanis, M., & Postmes, T. (2007). Two faces of anonymity: Paradoxical effects of cues to identity in CMC. *Computers in Human Behavior, 23*(2), 955–970.

Van Uden-Kraan, C. F., Drossaert, C. H., Taal, E., Seydel, E. R., & van de Laar, M. A. (2008). Self-reported differences in empowerment between lurkers and posters in online patient support groups. *Journal of Medical Internet Research, 10*(2), http://www.jmir.org/2008/2/e18/

Weinert, C., Cudney, S., & Winters, C. (2005). Social support in cyberspace: The next generation. *Computers, Informatics, Nursing, 23*(1), 7–15.

White, M. H., & Dorman, S. M. (2000). Online support for caregivers: Analysis of an Internet Alzheimer mailgroup. *Computers in Nursing, 18*(4), 168–176.

White, M. H., & Dorman, S. M. (2001). Receiving social support online: Implications for health education. *Health Education Research, 16*(6), 693–707.

Wright, K. B., & Bell, S. B. (2003). Health-related support groups on the Internet: Linking empirical findings to social support and computer-mediated communication theory. *Journal of Health Psychology, 8*, 39–54.

Ybarra, M. L., & Eaton, W. W. (2005). Internet-based mental health interventions. *Mental Health Services Research, 7*(2), 75–87.

CONCLUSION

IN COMPLETING THIS book, I think back to the day I began it. My intention was to update an earlier book (Kurtz, 1997), to make it more readable for group members and leaders, and to refocus that research on groups in mental health and addictions. The manuscript has grown in ways I did not imagine. The extra pages began with my decision to ground the work within the context of the recovery model, because recovery, after all, is the essence of self-help and support-community groups. In addition, I wanted to blend the recovery philosophy of the two fields of mental health and addictions.

Thinking and reading about recovery repeatedly brought me back to one simple idea and one word: hope. When follow-up to an acute case of mental illness or substance dependency proceeds, it should communicate hope for success in the recovery journey. And that is what recovery groups do so well. Such groups are peopled by members who have been recovering and who know how to recover; furthermore, they want to help others join them in that process of recovery without the need for a diagnostic label.

One morning, while finishing this manuscript, I found two important bits of news in the papers. The first was an article highlighting heroin overdoses reported in Washtenaw County where I live. The figures were going higher. Twenty-four young people had died of heroin overdoses in the past year in a county with 351,000 residents (Monson, 2014). There were pictures and comments by two main treatment center directors, Glynis Anderson and Jim Balmer. What I read next in the Wall Street Journal on the front page made me feel lucky to have them.

It was in-depth coverage of the shortage of mental health treatment facilities and personnel in the United States (Fields & Dooren, 2013). Out of 3,100 US counties, 55 percent had no available mental health treatment; 91 million people lived in an area where there was no mental health help. Of those practitioners who did serve in the rest of the counties, many did not accept insurance of any kind, and many others were so overbooked that they were taking no new patients. The reporters interviewed one psychiatrist who served one thousand patients at one time and did take insurance. This doctor's reimbursements by insurance companies had been pared so much that her income had fallen every year. She had now stopped practicing.

According to estimates, mutual-help and consumer-run groups and services already outnumber available traditional mental health and addiction treatment organizations (Goldstrom et al., 2006). These services are free for the most part, raising the question of how to make them available to even more consumers without destroying the very essence of what makes them valuable. The question is how treatment services can expand in such a way as to include long-term recovery resources in communities (White & Tuohy, 2013). With this question comes the plea for service providers and professionals to become more knowledgeable about and respectful of the grass-roots community of recovering people around them and make use of that community as part of an overall plan for care.

There are probably AA groups in all those 3,100 counties that have no mental health and addiction services; many of the same counties would also have NA groups, Al-Anon Family Groups, other twelve-step groups, non-twelve-step groups, mental health groups, and support groups. These groups do not do the same things professionals do, but they can give hope and support and experiential knowledge to people desperate for it. The richest nation cannot afford even minimal mental health and addiction treatment. But for people with both conditions, there is mutual aid, and it's free—because of the miracle that happened in New York City in 1935.

REFERENCES

Fields, G., & Dooren, J. C. (2013, December 21–22). For the mentally ill, finding treatment grows harder. *Wall Street Journal*, p. A1, p. A12.

Goldstrom, I. D., Campbell, J., Rogers, J. A., Lambert, D. B., Blacklow, B., Henderson, M. J., & Manderscheid, R. W. (2006). National estimates for mental health mutual support groups, self-help organizations, and consumer-operated services. *Policy in Mental Health Services Research, 33*(1), 92–103.

Kurtz, L. F. (1997). *Self-help and support groups: A handbook for practitioners*. Thousand Oaks, CA: Sage.

Monson, L. (2014, January). With a vengeance: The rise of prescription narcotics prompts the return of cheap, strong, plentiful heroin. *The Ann Magazine*, pp. 16–25.

White, W., & Tuohy, C. M. (2013). Recovery-oriented practice and the addictions professional: A systems perspective. *Advances in Addiction and Recovery (NAADAC)*, Summer, 22–23.

Acknowledgments

First, I thank my husband, Ernest Kurtz, for his editing, advice, and willingness to consult on every question I had as I worked on this manuscript. I especially appreciate his research on the content for chapter 13 on online groups. I also thank Bill White for his encouragement and support, for being willing to take the time to write a foreword with only two weeks' notice, and for his suggestions on chapter 11. I thank Tom Powell for his encouragement of this project and his review of the proposal and the manuscript. Keith Humphreys also took the time to review the proposal and make suggestions. I am grateful to Annette Smith for her comments on chapter 8 and permission to use her figure on AA Integration of Persons with a Low Degree of Affiliative Need and Group Dependency. I'm also grateful to Thomasina Borkman for her enthusiasm over the concept of the book and especially for her feedback on chapter 1. I owe Ruth Hollman a big debt of gratitude for her thorough review of the entire manuscript and her many suggestions. I am grateful to Brenda Hohman, Paul Boyer, John French, and Lin Jacobs for lending their stories. Thanks also to Pam Shultz for her comments on chapter 1. I thank Marilyn Wedenoja for her support and conversations about the concept of recovery in mental health and mental illness throughout the years I spent writing a proposal and the book itself. Finally, thanks also to my friends Mary Anna Bradshaw and Pat Kuessner for their encouragement over the years to just write.

Glossary

90/90 RULE: Ninety meetings in ninety days; a prescription often given to new members.

ARCO: Faces & Voices of Recovery Association of Recovery Community Organizations.

ASYNCHRONOUS ONLINE SITE : A participation website with e-mail exchanges.

CHAT ROOM: An Internet feature in which participants can send messages to one another in real time.

CLUBHOUSE MODEL: A mental health program in the community that has the characteristics of Fountain House in New York.

COMMUNITY MENTAL HEALTH CENTERS ACTS: Laws passed in 1963 allocating funds to build community mental health centers and in 1965 funding staff for those centers.

COMMUNITY SUPPORT PROGRAMS: Federal legislation in the 1970s that funded supportive housing, halfway houses, vocational training, transitional work, and services to the homeless.

CONSUMER/SURVIVOR: Someone who has received psychiatric treatment in the past.

DISEASE CONCEPT: The concept that addiction or mental disability is a response to a disease process mainly affecting the brain but also, in the case of alcohol addiction, other organs.

DUAL DIAGNOSIS: Having both an addiction to alcohol or another drug and a psychiatric disability.

EXPERIENTIAL KNOWLEDGE: The knowledge gained from personal experience with the condition.

FAIRWEATHER LODGE: A combination housing and employment program for long-term psychiatrically disabled people who live in the lodge and work in a business associated with the program.

FOUNTAIN HOUSE: The original clubhouse formed in New York in the 1940s, now serving 1,300 members.

GROUP COHESIVENESS: Having a sense of groupness and esprit de corps.

GROUP ENVIRONMENT: A concept formalized by Rudolph Moos in which elements of the group climate can be measured to show a group personality profile.

HELPER THERAPY PRINCIPLE: Those who help others are helped the most.

HOME GROUP: The group that the participant finds most appeals to his or her preferred meeting type and attends regularly; this term is used in twelve-step groups where individuals can attend many different groups in a week's time.

HUGHES ACT OF 1970: A law officially called the Comprehensive Alcohol Abuse and Alcoholism Prevention, Treatment, and Rehabilitation Act of 1970; introduced by Senator Harold Hughes of Oklahoma.

IDEAL TYPE: A construct that perfectly fits a definition; an extreme form of a concept used by sociologists in theories.

IDEOLOGY: How the group explains its members' common problems and what to do about them.

INSTILLATION OF HOPE: A group shares experiences of survival and successful recovery with newcomers and in that way instills hope.

LISTSERV: A group e-mail website in which participation occurs at different times; an asynchronous online site.

LURKING: Going to an online site where there is participation by others and not participating but merely observing.

MINDFREEDOM INTERNATIONAL: A coalition of consumer/survivor associations in Eugene, Oregon.

MINNESOTA MODEL: An alcoholism treatment model at Hazelden in Center City, Minnesota; the first-known formal treatment program that included peer helpers and AA meetings.

MUTUAL HELP OR MUTUAL AID: Used interchangeably with self-help; helping services between peers, either addicts or people with psychiatric labels.

NAMI: National Alliance on Mental Illness.

NCADD: National Council on Alcoholism and Drug Dependency.

NEUROPLASTICITY: The brain's ability to change with experience.

OXFORD GROUP: The First Century Christian group in the United States initiated by Frank Buchman, where the early AA founders first began meeting and from which they drew some of the ideas for AA. Not to be confused with the Oxford Movement in England.

OXFORD HOUSES: Homes for recovering people in which they form a mutual helping group among renters and support one another's recovery in the community.

PROCESS ADDICTION: A compulsive behavior that is not reinforced by drugs or alcohol; examples include gambling, sex, and food.

PSYCHOTHERAPY GROUP: A group led by a psychotherapist who controls interactions and interprets group dynamics or teaches a method of change and problem solving by the group.

RECOVERY CAPITAL: The resources needed to sustain recovery from an addiction or disability.

RECOVERY MODEL: A model of care that emphasizes hope and rehabilitation with the goal being a normal, satisfying life in spite of having a disability.

RECOVERY-SUPPORT SPECIALISTS: People who have a history of mental health or addiction treatment from which they have recovered enough to live a normal life, who are hired to work with recovering people in a nonclinical role. Similar to recovery coaches.

SELF-HELP ETHOS: A set of beliefs that emphasizes personal experience, empowerment, and democratic values.

SELF-HELP GROUP: A group of people with the same condition led by a peer, emphasizing a method of change in the self and the surroundings.

SENSE OF MATTERING: The feeling that others depend on us and are interested in us and concerned with our fate.

SOCIAL CAPITAL: The network of social connections among people that leads to mutually beneficial social cooperation.

SOCIAL WORLD: Boundaries are determined by interaction and communication, which transcend and cross over formal delineators of organization.

STRUCTURE: How the group is organized, its size, and its procedures in meetings.

SUPPORT GROUP: A group in which members have the same condition but are not seeking change, the purpose being support; may be led by a professional.

SYNCHRONOUS ONLINE SITE: A participation website in which discussion among users occurs in real time.

TRANSTHEORETICAL MODEL OF CHANGE: A change-readiness model from research on nicotine addiction.

UNIVERSALITY: Having a particular identity, a common problem, one core concern among group members.

WANA: We Are Not Alone, the loosely formed self-help group that came out of the state hospital in New York and formed the beginnings of Fountain House in 1948.

WORLDVIEW: Another way of defining how the group views the common problem and what should be done about it; similar to ideology.

Index

Page numbers in italics refer to materials in boxes or tables.

www.ingramcontent.com/pod-product-compliance
Lightning Source LLC
LaVergne TN
LVHW022208200926
848481LV00006B/1897